INFORMATION
AND
MEDICINE

Marsden S. Blois

INFORMATION AND MEDICINE

The Nature of Medical Descriptions

UNIVERSITY OF CALIFORNIA PRESS

Berkeley   Los Angeles   London

University of California Press
Berkeley and Los Angeles, California

University of California Press, Ltd.
London, England

Library of Congress Cataloging in Publication Data

Blois, Marsden S.
  Information and medicine.

  Bibliography: p. 273.
    1. Medicine—Data processing.   2. Information storage
and retrieval systems—Medicine.   I. Title.   [DNLM:
1. Information theory. 2. Computers. 3. Medicine.
W 26.5 B652i]
R858.B57 1984   610   83-24293
ISBN 0-520-04988-8

Printed in the United States of America

1 2 3 4 5 6 7 8 9

To Pat, Marsden, Byron, Stephen, Philip, and Mimi

Contents

Preface

During the past few decades the volume of medical knowledge has increased so rapidly that we are witnessing an unprecedented growth in the number of medical specialties and subspecialties. No longer is *internal medicine* viewed as the specialty it was only a generation ago, nor can the internist keep equally up to date in all its subspecialties. Medical educators are increasingly frustrated by the impossibility of communicating this mass of knowledge to the next generation of physicians. And absorbing this knowledge in the near absence of unifying or organizing principles taxes each new generation of medical students ever more severely. Finally, bringing this new knowledge to the aid of our patients in an economical and equitable fashion has stressed our system of medical care to the point where it is now declared to be in crisis. All these difficulties arise from the present, nearly unmanageable volume of medical knowledge, and the limitations under which humans can process information.

In the midst of all this, two remarkable new technologies have ripened—the digital computer and electronic data communications—to which physicians, medical educators, and health-system administrators have turned for help. Disappointingly, this aid has not been forthcoming as originally hoped, and obstacles which we regard as "informational" in nature continue to block our efforts at the very time when information technology is achieving its greatest successes. Why is this so?

If this paradox were fully understood, it would have been resolved long ago. Even now I believe that it is not some single barrier that bars our progress, and that it would be a mistake to look for one. Rather, there seems to be a number of issues that we have not seen fit to address seriously, and which, until we do, will continue to deflect our best efforts. One problem arises from our readiness to take technologies that have been developed for other purposes and apply them to medicine with little inquiry as to whether the problem environments are comparable. The transferal of techniques from other fields to medicine (ranging from the microscope to nuclear magnetic resonance imaging) has been enormously fruitful in the past, and in consequence the computer has tended to be looked upon as another instrument of general application to medicine. This may be a serious misconception.

The computer is a unique and subtle artifact. Instead of processing matter, converting energy from one form to another, or extending the power of our natural senses, it does one single thing—it manipulates symbols according to a set of instructions. And it does this superlatively well. Symbols, however, are tricky, nonmaterial things, though they must have a physical embodiment (magnetic spots, ink patterns, etc.) in order to be "processed." Symbols serve only a single purpose, to represent other things, and they are commonly regarded as containing information. Computers are built to process the symbols fed to them, in a manner prescribed by their programs, where the "meaning" of the symbols is known to the programmers but rarely to the program and never to the computer. Consequently, when we take the computer with its programs, which may have been originally developed for use in, say, applied mathematics, and apply it to medicine, we can transfer everything except the meaning.

We are obliged, as a consequence, to examine carefully what these application domains may have in common. In particular, we must ask whether they are *commensurable*. This, in my opinion, is done only rarely, and this omission is in part responsible for the relatively modest contribution of computers to medicine.

The reasons for the lack of progress in analyzing the nature of medical knowledge (which I would suggest is a necessary prerequisite to the proper utilization of computers in medicine) can be conjectured. Science and technology have their own dynamics and, once it was observed that the single thing computers do corresponds to one of the many things that brains do, a mystical relation between computers and brains was inferred. And, since the thing that computers do is frequently done by them more rapidly and accurately than it is by brains, there has been an irresistible urge to apply computers to medicine, but considerably less of an urge to attempt to understand where and how they can best be used.

These two different purposes continue to motivate workers in the field which we call medical information science, and contribute to the present uncertainty in defining its subject matter. One kind of activity is concerned with the application of a fairly well-understood technology to a poorly defined and complex problem environment, and can be regarded as engineering. The other is the attempt to understand why some of the problems of medicine are so ill defined and complex, and to search for structural features in medical knowledge. Some of these latter activities have been labeled "problem solving," "decision making," and "information retrieval," making them appear as clear and isolatable processes, which they are only rarely. Processes something like these are presumably of central importance to medicine but, like the last act of a play, they are not understandable without a knowledge of what has preceded them.

Singling out these processes as the proper goal of medical education remains perennially in fashion, along with decrying the "mere" teaching of facts. Yet what is the basis for distinguishing between the roles of substantive information (propositional knowledge) and process knowledge (skills) in medicine? An improved understanding of the structure of medical knowledge is needed if the interests of medical practice and medical education are to be served. This matter cannot simply be left to be reflected upon by others at their leisure; it lies at the heart of our dilemma.

The concerns of medical information science thus range from the designing and constructing of information systems (a useful but not especially interesting undertaking in the absence of a relevant theory) to the interesting but frequently unrewarded search for fundamental principles. In addition to the problems posed by such a breadth of goals, there is the concurrent need to train medical students (and older physicians as well) in the use of computers for "data and information management," while at the same time making them aware that there are as yet few theories of medicine that are of help in selecting such uses.

Since there is an abundant literature on *medical computing,* and virtually none on *medical information science* as a science, I began to teach a graduate course a few years ago dealing with some of the basic ideas of information science. For this purpose, I developed some sketchy notes and a few incompletely formulated concepts. Some of these have matured to the stage represented in this book. They are published under no illusion that they constitute a completed theory. Perhaps, at best, they afford some glimpses of what may lie beyond.

The studies underlying these essays extended over several years, and occupied two sabbatical leaves for which I am indebted to the University of California. My debts extend beyond this and include the Commonwealth Fund for a grant-in-aid, and the National Library of Medicine for assistance under a Special Project Grant (LM 00014). I am grateful to Dennis Marrian, Trinity College, Cambridge, and Karl Hausser, Max Planck Institute for Medical Research, Heidelberg, my gracious hosts during these two periods of study. Lotfi Zadeh, Gert Brieger, Roger Shannon, Mark Tuttle, Richard Sagebiel, David Bishop, David Sherertz, and Aaron Sicourel have generously provided me with both criticism and encouragement. The writing task could not have been completed without the help of Valerie Walters and Marina Gordillo, and the efficient and expert interventions of the University of California Press.

A part of chapter 7 is a revision of my earlier paper, "Clinical judgment and computers," which appeared in the *New England Journal of Medicine* (303:192-197, 1980), and is reprinted with the kind permission of the editor of the journal.

University of California, San Francisco   Marsden S. Blois
November 1983

1

Theories of Information

1.1 The Meanings of "Information"

We are concerned in this book with medical information but, if we are to achieve any insight into this subject, we must first clear away some of the underbrush that has grown up around the term *information*. Just what do we mean by "information"? This question may seem trivial; surely everyone knows what information is. It is the kind of commodity we can obtain at the information window at an airport, or something we need in order to accomplish a specific task. We probably assume that information, no matter how it is obtained, will possess such qualities as relevance, truthfulness, and usefulness. Information, as a commonsense notion, causes us little difficulty. However, all of this begs, but does not answer, the question.

If information is a thing or a commodity, as the commonsense view might have it, how is it possible for us to give information to others without having our own supply diminished? Why, having once given it to someone else, can we not later reclaim it? Or, since from time to time we are all given information we would just as soon not have, why can we not get rid of it? If information is a true commodity, do a hundred hearers of a lecture each acquire half as much as would only fifty? And does the larger audience deplete the lecturer twice as much? Such questions as these might raise awkward problems for proponents of the commodity view.

Because of questions such as these, alternative proposals have been made—that information may, after all, be a process rather than a commodity or, again, that it is something else, something altogether different. Certain concepts of information have received great emphasis from Claude Shannon's formulation of the mathematical theory of communications, and reveal his influence. We find information defined as "reduced uncertainty"[1] [7], or as "that which is used in decision making" [21]. Philosophers are fond of pointing out that often the first problem is to show that there *is* a problem. A little reflection at this point shows that defining "information" is a slippery matter.

It is commonplace nowadays to hear the expression "the information explosion." Professionals are finding it increasingly difficult to keep up with the advances being made in their fields, and as a result of this they continue to subdivide their fields into ever narrower specialties. The understanding (let alone the management) of our increasingly complex institutions requires more and more information, and all of us become aware of this when we are asked to prepare still more reports and to fill out still more forms. When the functioning of these institutions falters, it is frequently said that they do so because of a "communication" (i.e., information transfer) failure. In response to problems such as these, a considerable "information technology" has emerged over the past few decades.

It was realized at least a century before the first electronic digital computers were constructed that machines having these general capabilities could, in principle, not only process numbers (perform arithmetical computations) but also process information. When punched-card (Hollerith) machines and, later, electronic computers became available, certain basic processes, such as information storage and retrieval, and the sorting and listing of data, became feasible on a large scale. More recently, these processes have been extended to include text editing ("word processing"), typographical layout and composition, the graphical display of information, and data base creation, management, and inquiry. Research in the field known as "artificial intelligence" has resulted in computer programs that realistically imitate some of the processes that are thought to be characteristic of human cognition. Yet most of this progress has been accomplished with surprisingly little insight into what "information" is. Isaac Auerbach pointed out in 1974:

> The [data processing] business that I have described will be the third
> or fourth largest in the world by the end of another decade. We are
> spending a rather remarkable $13 billion a year in this industry. It is
> remarkable to observe how far we have progressed with so little true,
> scientific . . . understanding. [3]

The same criticism is echoed by Nicholas Belkin, an information
scientist engaged with the process of information retrieval:

> Although this [essay] is primarily concerned with explicitly proposed
> concepts of information, most work in information retrieval (IR) has
> managed somehow to proceed without any explicit statement [of
> what information is]. In particular, IR research and practice seem
> rarely to have considered this question at all. [8]

This need has continued to be unmet and has attracted surprisingly
little concern. M. Saito comments:

> We have tended to devote more time to constructing new systems
> than to the philosophical or theoretical . . . principles that underlie
> these applications, and [our] efforts have been empirical rather than
> fundamental. [107]

If computer and communication technologies have become the
most rapidly growing industries, it is because information processes consume such a large part of human activity, and not because we understand these processes well. In 1958, the economist
Fritz Machlup [75] estimated the scope of what he called the *information economy*. He defined this as that fraction of the national
economy concerned with the production, storage, and distribution
of information. Using the U.S. Department of Labor definitions
of various job categories, he estimated the effort consumed in
information processing for each type of occupation and, after
totaling his estimates, concluded that information-related activities accounted for approximately a third of the gross national
product.[2] Morris Collen and his associates analyzed the information-related processes in hospitals, and estimated that about a
third of a hospital's total operating budget was required to support informational activities [25]. But there is more than the economics of information at stake here. We view human beings as

information processors par excellence. In any attempt to understand human behavior, including such activities as understanding and reasoning, we continually need to invoke the notion of "information." Even though it might appear fruitless to seek an explanation of human behavior from purely informational considerations (although this has been attempted), it provides an important perspective from which to consider human activities.

1.2 Approaches to Concepts of Information

The first definition in Webster's unabridged dictionary for the verb *inform* (from L. *informare*) and now obsolete is *to give material form to,* and it is not until we get to the sixth definition that we find *to communicate knowledge to.* Similarly, for the noun *information,* the first definition is *an endowing with form* (obsolete), the second, *something received or obtained through informing* and, in fifth place we find *the process by which the form of an object of knowledge is impressed upon the apprehending mind so as to bring about the state of knowing.* At the outset it is suggested to us that information has something to do with form, and that this may have been central to its ancient meaning. The dictionary also tells us that information is a thing—the thing "received or obtained through informing"—but it then goes on to state that it is a process. In the end we are given little basis for deciding whether information is a thing or a process. Since "information" does not have a single, clear meaning, the reader might conclude that there is no single, satisfactory theory of information. That is indeed the case.

What should we expect of a theory of information? Belkin has proposed a test to be met by a theory of information if it is to be useful in information science [8]:

1. It must refer to information within the context of purposeful, meaningful communication.
2. It should account for information as a social communication process among human beings.
3. It should account for information's being requested or desired.
4. It should account for the relationship between information and state of knowledge (of generator and recipient).

5. It must be generalizable beyond the particular case.
6. It must offer a means for prediction of the effect of information.

Concepts of "information" are employed in disciplines ranging from philosophy and physics to psychology. These different concepts bear the stamp of their fields of origin. They are commonly specific to a particular set of phenomena, and they seem narrow when compared with the range of phenomena requiring explanation. When information is taken to be the subject of human communication, a satisfactory concept of information must span activities ranging from the thought processes of someone who picks up a telephone to place a call through all the intervening workings of the technical machinery to the changes in the mind of the person who receives the call. When this overall process is broken down and analyzed piecemeal, the resulting theories of information tend to become "theories of speakers," "theories of communication channels," "theories of listeners," and "theories of decision makers." In order to make any progress, we must consider examples of what people seem to mean when they use the term "information." The most frequent *specialized* use of this term is one encountered in mathematics and engineering and, if one looks up "information" or "information theory" in a library catalog, the majority of citations will be found in these categories. It is essential, therefore, to consider this body of work briefly before proceeding to more general matters.

1.3 Information As a Subject of Engineering and Mathematics

One major line of inquiry originated at the beginning of this century in the field of radio engineering, picked up support from studies in physics in the thirties, forties, and fifties, and resulted in a "theory of information" in the United States, and a "communication theory" in Great Britain. This early uncertainty about a suitable name for the theory must have reflected an underlying doubt about the nature of the subject matter. We will see shortly how these doubts arose. As an engineering subject, this particular theory of information plays a central role in telecommunications and computer science and, as a by-product, it has resulted in the development of a separate branch of mathematics. Beyond this, it has introduced a new vocabulary to the world of science and a new way of viewing things. Thus we now find such statements as "... it is certain that the conceptual connection between information and the second law of thermodynamics is now firmly established" [128]. Let us see what this statement means.

In the early days of radio telegraphy, H. Nyquist [91] and K. Kuepfmueller [63] independently pointed out that, in order to transmit signals at some chosen rate, a calculable bandwidth or frequency range was required. This law was reformulated in a more general form by R. V. L. Hartley in 1927 [57]. Hartley's law states that, in order to transmit a specified message, a certain fixed product (bandwidth x time) is required. If one wishes to transmit the same message in half the time, a communication channel with twice the bandwidth must be provided. Hartley's law is basic and pervasive. If we seek higher-fidelity voice communication, we can obtain it only by providing (at increased expense) a greater bandwidth. This is all a matter of physics.

In formulating any theory in natural science, and stating it in mathematical form, it is first necessary to create an abstraction of some real situation. One must then state explicitly what the different terms of this abstraction represent. It was clear to Hartley that, during a communication, *something,* in addition to matter or energy, was being transferred from an originator to a receiver. Hartley decided that this something was "information," and the title of his paper became "Transmission of Information." Hartley's procedure was to *define* information in terms of the process of selecting particular symbols (such as a Morse code sequence) from a list of possible symbols in order to create the desired message. He recognized that not all the sequences of symbols that could be chosen would be meaningful or understandable, so he ignored any "meaning" that the message might have as being irrelevant. His theory consequently treated all symbol combinations as being on an equal footing. A sequence of letters, whether chosen purposefully or at random would, according to Hartley's definition, contain information. From this point on, Hartley's development (and later developments derived from it) diverges from the sense of "information" in which our interest lies.

A collection of symbols, whether assembled purposefully, gathered carelessly, or mixed together randomly, does in fact contain something. Hartley called it "information" and set about deriving a measure for it. Since his measure is equally applicable to sense or nonsense, his information content is purely a technical one, and of limited applicability to the broader subject of human communication. He proceeded to point out that a message of *n* words (or symbols) taken from a list of *N* words, can be selected in N^n different ways. He then reasoned that the "information content" (*H*) of a message (which he defined as the probability of its having been chosen from the set of all possible messages of equal length) can be expressed in the form $H = n \log N$. Commenting upon Hartley's definition of "information," Colin Cherry has commented:

> In a sense, it is a pity that the mathematical concepts stemming from Hartley have been called "information" at all. The formula for (*H*) is really a measure of one facet only of the concept of information. [21]

Hartley's legacy thus becomes a concept of information that excludes meaning. Since he explicitly defined information content in terms of the probability of drawing a particular signal sequence (message) from a set or repertoire of possible sequences and, at the same time, denied the relevance of meaning, he unwittingly set a trap for us. Yehoshua Bar-Hillel has commented that psychologically it is almost impossible not to make the shift from one sense of information (information = signal sequence) to a different sense (information = what is expressed by the signal sequence) [6]. This use of the word *information* to include not only meaningful messages but meaningless ones as well was destined to be extended still further.

1.4 The Hartley-Shannon-Weaver View of Information

The extension of Hartley's ideas to include the effects of noise and coding procedures upon communication channel capacity was carried out by Shannon and published in an influential paper in 1948 [112]. Shannon has also cautioned against the application of this theory to processes involving meaning: "In any case, meaning is quite irrelevant to the problem of transmitting the information. ... Thus in information theory, information is thought of as a choice of one message from a set of possible messages" [114].

In order to distinguish between these two uses of the same word, let us call what Hartley and Shannon are measuring "S-information" (as a mnemonic for Shannon-information), and what humans exchange, which has the effect of changing another person's knowledge, "H-information" (for human-information). These concepts of information differ, and it is useful to make their differences explicit.

Shannon's aim had been an analysis of the effect of noise and coding procedures on communication-channel capacity (for the transmission of S-information). The problem of noise and the process of coding are not essential in appreciating the difference between our two senses of information, but Hartley's "selection" or "statistical" view of information is. In order to be able to think about channel capacity, it is necessary to be able to conceive of whatever it is that is passing over the channel. For this purpose, Shannon began with Hartley's definition of information as something arising from the selection of message elements from a set of such elements, and he applied Hartley's measure to the result of this process.

Instead of using a term like *message* to encompass everything communicated, from pulse patterns to handwritten letters, let us adopt a more specific terminology. We will call the messages or signals that, upon receipt by a mechanical device, result in the performance of a specific act or series of acts, *instructions*. When we press the *A* key on a teletype, it is an instruction that is transmitted to the receiving device. When we dial someone's telephone number, the pulse train (or tone sequence) which is transmitted to the central switching equipment is a set of such instructions. And what is encoded in a nucleic acid sequence and directs the synthesis of a particular protein is a set of instructions.

When we regard this kind of selection as involving "information," we open the way to an extended series of usages of this word, such as: DNA contains "information," a key to a tumbler lock contains "information" or, even, a socket wrench contains "information." It is obvious that each of these things possesses something that arises from its shape or pattern, which permits it to perform a specific operation. Calling this something "selection power" or S-information avoids committing ourselves to the idea that it is identical with, or even resembles, what humans exchange when they communicate. And S-information can always be measured in terms of its "selection power," which is readily computed from Hartley's formula.[3]

If we distinguish between the constraints imposed upon a human in composing a message (perhaps idly choosing between chocolate or vanilla) and the deterministic behavior shown by a machine, such as a teletype, we come much closer to understanding what it is that Shannon is measuring. In selecting a letter of the English alphabet (by drawing letters out of a hat, for example), we have a well-defined set of possible letters from which a choice can be made, and the Hartley-Shannon measure is readily applied to the resulting collection. We do not have to worry about what this selection might mean; the measure is operational. But if we think of selecting individual English words, as in the composition of a telegram, the application of this measure immediately raises difficulties. How many English words are there for us to choose from? Where are we to find this set of ''all possible'' English words? We could not even address an envelope if we could use only the words in the dictionary. What are we to do about the newly coined ones, which enter the language continuously? Are we to allow informal or casual names, or nicknames or place names? And what counts as an ''English'' word? Finally, when we come to sequences of words, how could we conceivably measure the set of all possible sentences? How could we begin to go about designing a procedure for enumerating them? Hartley's measure at this point fails to be operational at all.

Warren Weaver believes the human communication problem to consist of three levels:

Level A. How accurately can the symbols of communication be transmitted? (The technical problem.)

Level B. How precisely do the transmitted symbols convey the desired meaning? (The semantic problem.)

Level C. How effectively does the received meaning affect conduct in the desired way? (The effectiveness problem.)

Referring to Shannon's theory, he then goes on to say,

> . . . the mathematical theory of the engineering aspects of communication . . . admittedly applies in the first instance only to Level A. . . . But a larger part of the significance comes from the fact that the analysis at Level A discloses that this level overlaps the other levels more than one could possibly naively suspect. Thus, the theory of Level A is at least to a significant degree, also a theory of levels B and C. [114]

Since Hartley (and Shannon, both in his original paper [112] and later as well [113] had stipulated that the theory of level A is irrelevant to the problem of meaning, one may wonder how Weaver reached this conclusion.

Consider the strings of symbols that teletype machines send and receive. Pressing the *A* key on the keyboard of the sending machine sends out a unique train of pulses, which the receiving machine accepts as the instruction to print the letter *A*. If the next letter typed were a *T*, the teletype would print this too, without knowing that it had just produced a word. And if the transmission continued and produced *AT ONCE*, none of the hardware would experience any sense of urgency. We can indicate this overall process with reference to the organizational levels involved (a representation that will be more fully developed in chapter 3):

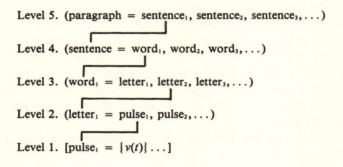

Level 5. (paragraph = sentence$_1$, sentence$_2$, sentence$_3$, . . .)

Level 4. (sentence = word$_1$, word$_2$, word$_3$, . . .)

Level 3. (word$_1$ = letter$_1$, letter$_2$, letter$_3$, . . .)

Level 2. (letter$_1$ = pulse$_1$, pulse$_2$, . . .)

Level 1. [pulse$_1$ = {$v(t)$} . . .]

Figure 1.1

If we were to examine the physical communication channel itself (level 1 in fig. 1.1), all that we could note would be voltage variations occurring over time. A voltage flowing for a specific unit of time makes a pulse, and a particular sequence of pulses, together with the spaces between them, may be assigned to a particular letter or keyboard function. The sequence of pulses at level 1 are thus interpreted as letters at level 2 (fig. 1.1). That is as far as the teletype machine can go. It can contribute nothing further to the communication process. Hartley (and his predecessors) showed that, as a matter of physics, these pulses could not be transmitted arbitrarily fast—either over a pair of wires or by means of traveling electromagnetic waves—and that the product (bandwidth x time) sets the limit. Shannon's extension of Hartley's work deals with the efficient assignment of pulse patterns to represent letters (coding), the effect of intervening noise pulses that might occur in the channel, and the use of redundancy to overcome the errors introduced by noise. Shannon's theory is a theory of levels 1 and 2 in this figure (which correspond to Weaver's level A).

The next step, however—putting together letters to form words (going from level 2 to level 3, in fig. 1.1—is governed by the dictionary of the language being used and the human user's linguistic customs. These constraints are not imposed upon the teletype system (Shannon's theory is not a theory of dictionaries or of words) but upon the human creator of the message. The originator of a message is not at liberty to spell words arbitrarily if he wishes to be understood. Words in turn become more powerful when they can be arranged to form sentences (level 3 to level 4), and this process is largely determined by the syntax of the language. This too is a set of constraints imposed solely upon the human originator and has no effect upon the machine. Shannon's theory is not a theory of grammar. Sentences can be further arranged to construct paragraphs, so that a message creator is able to emphasize and distinguish topics. This too is a wholly human process, and is virtually unconstrained, being determined only by the skill of the human message creator and the context in which communication occurs. The reader will have noted that, as we move from one descriptive level to a higher one, certain systematic changes set in. In the next chapters we will find that these changes are characteristic of hierarchical organizations, and that they profoundly affect our ability to communicate.

Weaver's proposal that the Shannon theory propagates upward in this hierarchy, and contributes to the explanation of the events occurring at higher levels, seems difficult to reconcile with the foregoing analysis. Though it is clearly applicable to the transition from level 1 to level 2, how, for example, could this theory go further and account for the spelling of words? It might well say something about the random process by means of which noise in a transmission channel can distort a transmitted word into an incorrectly received one, or it might even provide the basis for an automatic means for correcting certain kinds of errors. But the mechanical system cannot detect, as a human might, the receipt of an inappropriately chosen word. A human is able to detect such errors since, unlike a machine, words and symbols make sense or nonsense, and it is the meaning and context that count. However, the Shannon theory, by excluding meaning, cannot deal with context and is uninfluenced by it. Although there was much optimism in the 1950s that Shannon's theory would contribute to the understanding of human communication, there has been little evidence produced since then that this is possible. We are thus left with separate theories—theories of channels, syntactic rules, semantics —and, above all, with our attempts to explain what moves humans to communicate.

It may be helpful to recount this process by proceeding in the opposite direction. We have examined the process of printing out a sentence or paragraph in terms of what a receiving teletype machine does when it receives a string of electrical pulses. When humans communicate they begin with no such things as electrical pulses. The *origin* of our messages lies far above the top level of figure 1.1. Our initial disposition or intention to produce an utterance or sentence arises in a particular situation and because we have a certain purpose or expectation. Only after these dispositions or intentions have attained some coherence are we even moved to communicate. Then we may proceed to form utterances or sentences. Human communication enters the picture from the top of this diagram, and a variety of prelinguistic processes will have already been completed before the matter of sentence formation arises. Only after our communicative plans have been shaped in some detail do we construct sentences.

The next problem is that of converting an intention or desire into a linear sequence of sounds or words. That linearization is involved here (in process as well as in result) becomes evident when we must pause while speaking or writing to think of an appropriate word. Natural language is sequential, although there seems little evidence that all of thought is.[4] And of course nowhere in the process of speaking do we think in terms of letters. An illiterate person is perfectly able to speak. Only after we have reduced our thoughts to a sequence of words, and then only when using written language, do letters themselves even enter into the communication process. The activities of a teletype machine enter at the bottom level shown in figure 1.1, whereas those of a human enter at vastly higher levels, which are not even implied by the diagram.

There would seem to be a call for at least two criticisms, then, of Weaver's explication of Shannon's theory. One is with respect to the idea of "selection" when it is applied to human communication. This concept was expressed by Shannon when he remarked that, "The significant aspect is that the actual message is one selected from a set of possible messages" [18]. The widespread notion that the information content of a statement is to be measured not by what *was* said but by what *could have been* said raises more problems than it solves. Although this is an important concept in physics and leads to a useful measure of the selection power of a telephone number, or as a measure of selection power in DNA, it offers little insight into human communications. Donald MacKay, an early contributor to communication theory, has commented that the difficulty of measuring this "set of possible messages" has impeded the application of this form of "information theory" in the manner originally anticipated [78]. Beyond the matter of difficulty is that of measurability, even in principle.

A second objection to the selection concept arises when we note that, if two people were to have sets of "potential messages" differing in size (which would appear to be the usual case) and if each were to state "It is raining outside," this same utterance would (under the Hartley-Shannon theory) have two different measures of information content. Which one are we to choose? Applying the theory in this manner (if we could) would seem to measure properties of message creators rather than of messages.

It is sometimes asserted (according to this theory) that information is a measure of the "surprise value" of a message. Under this view, "The dog bit the man" and "The man bit the dog" have been claimed to have unequal information content. Yet each statement draws attention to two objects and to a clear relation between them. They would appear to be symmetrical, though no one would quarrel with the claim that the second of these has the greater "surprise value" or is the more newsworthy. It's just that these properties may have little to do with "information content." Whether or not someone is surprised by a message depends upon his expectations, and his personal knowledge of the world. The application of this notion thus leads to an information measure that measures properties of the hearer of a message, and not to the message itself.

Human communication goes far beyond simple message exchange and it might be expected to display still other features. A telephone call received in the middle of the night has its own message beyond that of the content of the call. Understanding even the simple statement "I won't do it" requires an appreciation of context, whether it is said in acquiescence or in refusal.

The Hartley-Shannon theory deals with the "closed" communications of machines in which the communicated symbols are the objects of interest, and where the symbols are considered apart from meaning. When our interest is specifically in the meaning and we attach secondary importance to the symbols used to convey it, this theory can give us little help.

1.5 Other Concepts of Information

A viewpoint developed from the perspective of decision theory by B. J. Whittemore and M. C. Yovits is that "... information is data of value in decision making" [138]. This may appear to be a fairly narrow definition, but the authors proceed to define decision making as "... purposeful activity of intelligent behavior." The role of information in the decision-making process is then asserted to be the reduction of uncertainty. The model they employ considers the decision maker to be at any given moment in a particular "decision state," which is characterized by his knowledge of courses of action, possible outcomes, goals, and states of nature. A measure of the uncertainty associated with the decision state is then derived.

One difficulty with this measure, as Belkin [8] has pointed out, is that there is no procedure provided for carrying out the necessary measurements. But there are other difficulties, as well. Before turning to these, we might look into the reasons Yovits gives for undertaking his program. After observing (correctly, as we have argued) that the Hartley-Shannon concept, by disregarding meaning, provides too restrictive an approach to the nature of information for it to be useful in information science, Whittemore and Yovits comment: "At the other extreme, the treatment of information to be synonymous with knowledge appears to be far too broad to lead to meaningful and useful principles" [138]. Without further consideration of this "other extreme," they adopt a different position by defining information to be *data of value in decision making*. They point out that, of Weaver's three levels of information (p. 9), the Shannon theory applies only to the first level, and deals with what Weaver called the "technical problem."

They identify their own theory with Weaver's third level, which is concerned with the "effectiveness problem." This, it is stated, "deals with the effectiveness of information—that is, how information, once received and understood, is utilized."

Thus Shannon's theory of information stops just short of coming to grips with the fact that H-information has meaning, and he thereby confines himself in principle to the first level. Whittemore and Yovits, on the other hand, begin with the third of Weaver's levels, and again, by ignoring meaning, proceed directly to the matter of effectiveness. In order to develop measures of the effectiveness of information, they formulate three hypotheses which, they state, are necessary for a "generalized information system":

1. Information is data of value in decision making.
2. Information gives rise to observable effects.
3. Information feedback exists so that the decision maker will adjust his model for later similar decisions.

Hypothesis 1 is to be understood in the restrictive sense. For something to be information, it must be "data of value in decision-making." Thus they go on to state, curiously, that "If information is received, but never used or applied to a subsequent decision, then its effect does not exist and it cannot be measured." This implies that there may be two kinds of information—one that is capable of being understood but which is not acted upon (a measurable or observable "effect" does not exist), and one that is both understood and results in some overt behavioral change. The first kind of information is thus excluded from their theory, which becomes a theory of information "when it is used in decision making." Unless decision making is regarded in some extended sense as being equivalent to cognition generally, their definition would not appear to include much of the information that is involved in telling jokes, or writing textbooks, novels, or poems, activities in which one would suppose Weaver's "effectiveness" might readily be judged.

Hypothesis 2 thus confers a peculiar status upon the kind of information that is received and understood but is not acted upon. It would seem that we commonly pass on information to others that cannot be used (or produce an effect) until appropriate circumstances arise. Whittemore and Yovits might be interpreted as saying that information regarding an antidote cannot exist until a poisoning has occurred. Meanwhile, what are we to call this thing that is received through language, that is understood, and that forms a part of our knowledge? If we never act upon it, can it then be said that it never existed or that we never received it? Or, if we do act upon it, perhaps only later when the appropriate circumstances arise, does this curious something only then become information? Their second hypothesis, that information must give rise to some observable behavioral change, is reminiscent of a stimulus-response view of cognition. If this is the case, their argument becomes subject to many of the cogent criticisms made by Noam Chomsky in his review of B. F. Skinner's *Verbal Behavior* [22].

Propositions that regard idle thoughts or passing fancies as decision processes suffer from still other difficulties. There is, first and foremost, the matter of decomposability. We must ask whether some overall process, like getting out of bed or shaking hands with someone, can be broken down into a discrete series of primitive subprocesses, each of which in turn can be represented in terms of decisional primitives. One of the difficulties with this view is that, if we are at a particular stage of such a process, what in fact can the next step be? Can such a thing even be defined? As with Zeno's problem of Achilles and the tortoise, are we doomed to pursue an infinite sequence of intermediate states before we reach a decision or complete an action [105]? Or is it rather the case that our cognitive processes (like Achilles' race) are completed in a single continuous action?

The suggestion that the information content of a message is somehow related to the magnitude of the change in the knowledge state of someone who understands the message is an appealing one. It seems consistent with the proposal (which we will consider shortly) that the information content of a statement could be measured by the number of assertions that it makes about the world. It would appear that the greater the number of assertions about some state of affairs that a statement or message makes, the greater the changes in a hearer's knowledge.[5] Yet this view is not without its own difficulties. A message or statement is a public and objective thing that can be studied by various observers. An individual's state of knowledge, in contrast, is a private matter not entirely accessible even to its owner. Neither messages nor knowledge states (if there are such things) are at present susceptible to such formalization, but the prospects of being able to understand messages would seem more promising than the prospects of being able to understand knowledge states. If this possibility did not exist, linguistics could have only the most limited of aims. It is a common experience that various observers will describe an object or event in quite different ways, and yet convey substantially the same meaning. Although their various descriptions have different surface structures, it is at a deeper level that the information content of such descriptions must be measured.

I have considered several propositions about what "information" may be. As it turned out, our inquiry seems to have been more concerned with what it is not. I shall now turn to the task of developing an affirmative notion of information, using the particular instance of descriptive information as it is employed in medicine.

2

Problems with "Information"

2.1 What Does Information Do?

Up to now, I have discussed what information *is*. Now, let us talk about what information *does,* which may prove to be easier.

Once we have become informed about something, we are never quite the same as we were before. Even after we have forgotten the details, we retain a memory of once having known something about the matter in a general way. What do we mean when we say that we have been "informed" about some matter or that we have "received information"? The intuitive meaning seems to be that our knowledge of some state of affairs in the world has been altered. After receiving new information, we no longer view the world in exactly the same manner as we did before. A common alteration is the *addition* of some fragment of knowledge previously absent. We can always learn something new. Another is the *correction* of our earlier beliefs ("Tom Brown's telephone number is 333-6141, not 333-6411") or the *revision* or *updating* ("The vice-premier of China is now in London") of previous knowledge.

These readily recognized actions involve two elements, one is called information, and the other, knowledge. We imply thereby that there must be a process by means of which information is able in some way to alter knowledge. The question of how knowledge is represented in minds (or brains) is one that must be left for cognitive psychologists and neurobiologists to answer in the future. So, too, is an explanation of how we are able to alter this representation through introspection or, actually, what "understanding" consists of. We readily recognize that we have received information in the past that we did not grasp completely at the time, but which became clear to us only later. This may occur with surprising abruptness (the ah-HA! or Eureka! phenomenon). Although these matters are little understood, we can hope to refine the meanings we attach to the words we need by using them. The mere use of terms such as *information* and *knowledge* cannot explain them, yet it is only through the use of them that we can begin to clarify the meanings they have for us, and to recognize the circumstances in which we can properly employ them.

We will begin, then, with the commonsense notion that there is in our minds (brains) a record of all we have experienced. This record may suffer from incompleteness, lapses of memory, faults in organization, failures in understanding, and from certain outright pathologies. Nevertheless, it is all we have that links us with our own past, provides us with our identity, and underlies our expectations of the future. Whatever its limitations, it is the source of our recallable thoughts and much of our mental activity generally. This record may be regarded as our "cognitive map" of the world but, whatever it is called, it must include a representation of our knowledge of the world, including ourselves and our own mental processes. More accurately, this representation *is* our knowledge. This representation, or cognitive map, undergoes almost continuous change—ordinarily in only small details—so long as there is any mental activity at all. It may also change under pathological conditions, such as trauma or disease. Certain of these changes that take place in our knowledge, and the ones with which we will be occupied here, are induced by perceived changes in the world.

We now come to a primary concept of the connection between the world and our minds: the concept of *perception*. By this we denote the collection of processes set into motion by the receipt of stimuli upon our sense organs (or, more generally, upon our bodies as a whole) and the subsequent integrating activities of the central nervous system, which result in awareness. Fortunately, not all the stimuli arriving at our sensory surfaces have this result —we can learn how to ignore distracting noises. Nor are all instances of awareness initiated by sense perception. Under conditions of sensory deprivation, for example, we will continue to have thoughts, and we may become aware, through reflection, of circumstances of which we had previously been oblivious. Much of what we know about the world, and *all* that we have learned from our personal experiences, is acquired through the action of the world upon our bodies. It is equally clear that not *all* our knowledge of the world is acquired through direct experience, since we learn of things vicariously from the reported experiences of other people. Whether or not we have a priori knowledge of things that we have not perceived is a question that will not detain us here.

All of us appear to have certain kinds of acquired knowledge which is embedded so deeply that it cannot be made wholly explicit. This type of knowledge has been called "knowing how" knowledge, and would include "knowing how" to ride a bicycle and "knowing how" to swim. This kind of knowledge is frequently difficult, and may be impossible, to articulate fully. It may be beyond the reach of introspection or recall, and portions of it may be "innate," as Michael Polanyi has argued [97]. It appears that we know more than we think we know. This innate or personal kind of knowledge is to be contrasted with the "knowing that" sort—for example, that Charles de Gaulle was a former president of France. Here we either know something or we do not, and we can usually tell the difference. Knowledge of this second type is most closely related to the concept of information that we will be developing. For us to be able to describe things or to understand the descriptions created by others, it is this readily communicable kind of knowledge that counts.

It would be risky, however, for us to begin by assuming that knowledge exists in only certain restricted or fixed kinds of "knowing." The distinction we have just suggested cannot be taken as a sharp one, and these two types of knowledge might better be thought of as the extremes of a continuum rather than as disjoint categories. Ordinary experience tells us that this must be so. When we carry out an act requiring some special or "expert" knowledge—say in preparing an unusual dish for the first time—this special knowledge alone does not suffice unless it is supported by commonsense knowledge, by knowing where to find the eggs and milk, for instance. And for the enterprise to succeed, we require the underlying innate or personal knowledge of how to break eggs, or how to use an eggbeater successfully. Though it is helpful to be able to refer to notions like "expert," "commonsense," and "innate" knowledge, it may be impossible in an actual situation to say where one of these ends and another begins. It is this continuity of cognitive performance that resists our attempts to decompose it or describe it formally.

The medical enterprise is commonly regarded as one that is "information-intensive." The observations that physicians carry out, the decisions they make, and the acts they perform depend upon information processes in an important way. The distinction (to the extent that this is meaningful) between "knowing how" and "knowing that" has a particular relevance to medicine. "Knowing how" includes much of the observational, verbal, and motor skills of the physician, and of this kind of knowing a great deal may be difficult to articulate, or may be impossible to explain at all. These skills play a vital role in the practice of medicine. They are difficult to teach, and they are responsible for medical education being in large part an apprenticeship. The "knowing that" kind of knowledge is more objective; it is public, and it can be classified, gathered into textbooks, and organized into lectures. This is also the kind of knowledge that is being dealt with increasingly through the use of computers. This distinction is useful in attempting to understand the difficulties involved both in medical education and in the proper selection of roles for computers in medicine.

Bertrand Russell divided knowledge in yet another way. He called knowledge acquired through our direct perception of some state of affairs in the world—we see that it is raining outside, or we hear the doorbell ringing—"knowledge by acquaintance." He spoke of a second kind of knowing, one of greater interest to us here, as "knowledge by description." This is the knowledge of the world we receive indirectly through the reports of others who may themselves have acquired it through direct perception. It is to be conceded that knowledge by description would be denied to us as well were it not for perception but, in this case, it is the *description* of a state of affairs that we perceive and not the state of affairs itself. Russell's two types of knowledge play rather different roles; knowledge by acquaintance would seem to have the greater survival value in the context of evolutionary biology. This is the predominant type in beasts. Acquisition of knowledge by description requires a developed system of communication and, in its more advanced forms, it is a distinctively human affair.

Most important, a description of an object or an event has an existence that is external to the describer and, in the case of a recorded description, has permanence as well. This type of knowledge is therefore a prime driving force in the processes of social and cultural evolution. When knowledge is once made objective by its disclosure in public, it becomes an object of study for other minds. Procedures of verification become possible, methods for distinguishing belief from true knowledge emerge, the notion of consensus appears, and the possibility of science comes into being. We shall adopt, then, the concept of "information" as a "thing" which, upon receipt, alters our knowledge—alters the mental representation we have, which is our map of the world.

2.2 The "Thing" View of Information

Information can be communicated in many different message forms: spoken language, sign language, body language, pictures, and maps, to mention only a few. We will begin by considering natural language. Spoken language is believed to have become conventionalized and well developed long before written language appeared. The differences between them are important and deep. But we will first consider a matter that involves them both: the question of when an utterance or a written message can be said to be meaningful. When can something be said "to be" information?

In his Tarner Lectures, Alfred North Whitehead tells us that "all thought has to be about things" [136]. This may sound vaguely like something we learned in grammar school—that sentences have subjects, and that it is the subject that the sentence is about. This idea is a useful starting point, but it does not explain enough. We need to inquire further into both the "thing" and the "aboutness" that are involved. Suppose someone tells us that "grass is green." This utterance says something about something, it is understandable, and it certainly conveys information. But in doing so it accomplishes two quite different ends. The utterance brings a thing, grass, to our attention, and it then asserts a property of it. It is this combination of a thing and some claim about the thing that is required if information is to be successfully transferred.

If someone were to utter, *totally out of context,* "grass" or "green," we would say that these utterances were not complete messages. They are, in fact, not messages at all but only message fragments. I would argue further that the utterance "grass" or "green" does not convey information, since neither one can change our state of knowledge. They do not describe, question, or command. Our state of knowledge *would be* changed, of course, by our direct perception of both the speaker's moving lips and the noises he is making. We would then know that John Jones said "grass," just as we would know that John Jones said "yok," if that had been his utterance. But neither utterance in itself could change our state of knowledge about the world, since nothing has been said about it. Such attempts at message formation do not convey information. If, in contrast, John Jones had said "grass is green," we would have our state of knowledge changed to reflect the fact that he made the utterance (as evidenced by our perception of his vocal efforts), and we would know (if we did not already) that grass is green.

We might suspect from this example that there could be many utterances or bits of text so fragmentary in nature that they could not meet the test of being (or containing) information according to our definition. Our suspicion would be well founded, and the reason for it has been long recognized. As Russell put it, "... there is a basis in traditional logic which assumes that every proposition has a subject and a predicate. According to this view, every fact consists in something having some property"[1] [104]. In order for an utterance or written message to convey information, it must first draw a listener's (or reader's) attention to a particular thing, and then assert a property of it. This condition—which we will call the *completeness condition*—is necessary but by no means sufficient for the successful transfer of information.

In applying the completeness test, it should be noted that it is applicable only to context-free situations.[2] For example, both of the isolated utterances "grass" and "green" would be completely informative if given in response to the command "Give me an example of something that is green" or the question "What is the color of grass?" But context may be provided by nonlinguistic means as well, and this is common. If we were to come upon a person splashing around in the middle of a lake and at the same time crying "Help!" this single word would be a fully informative message, given the context. But a roadside sign displaying only this single word would surely not be. In written communications especially, the message must be self-explanatory to the intended recipient. It must meet the completeness condition if it is to be understood.

For the sake of convenience we have considered examples expressed in natural language, but it can be seen that the completeness requirement applies to information transfer processes more generally. Consider the case of highway signs. One labeled "Berkeley," and displaying an arrow pointing to a freeway off-ramp, conveys a complete message and is understandable. One marked only "Berkeley," or one with only an arrow, might not convey a complete message in the absence of further clues. Signs such as "55 MPH" and "STOP" are readily understood because these usages have become conventionalized within the context of highway signs. But a sign reading "OUCH!" would be meaningless, since this form is unconventional and there would be no context.

2.3 Things and Attributes

The completeness condition—that a message or utterance must draw attention to at least one thing, and assert at least one property of it if it is to contain information—would seem to be a minimal and necessary condition. "Grass is green" satisfies this condition, and this message is informative. If this is the minimum condition, is there then any upper limit to the number of things and attributes that a message can contain? Clearly not. The sentence "Rome is the capital of Italy, Paris of France, . . ." could be extended to great and awkward length, be completely grammatical, and be readily understood. There are no logical or linguistic limits to how much we can say about the world, only the practical ones of time and energy. These are what brought to an end the efforts of Tristram Shandy, who began to write his autobiography in the greatest possible detail and, after a year's writing, had only described the first day of his life.

Instead of attempting to say everything, we say only those things that will serve our purposes in particular situations. Human communication (as with most biological processes) represents a compromise between economy and reliability. In creating our utterances or sentences, we are free to name other things or to assert additional attributes until we are satisfied with our construction. Thus, if it serves our purpose, we may assert a number of attributes about a single thing: "Grass is green, and is eaten by sheep, cows, deer, ... " Or we may call attention to a number of things about which we assert a single attribute: "Grass, frogs, dollar bills, ... are green."

In these extended utterances we refer to increasing portions of the world, and we expect them to induce correspondingly greater changes in the knowledge states of our hearers. We expect that these extended utterances contain more information. It appears, for example, that the sentences "Grass is green," "Grass is green, and is eaten by cows," and "Leaves and grass are green, and are eaten by cows and sheep" contain increasing amounts of information since the number of things or attributes increases, and the sentences say increasingly more about the world.

In this intuitive view of the matter of information content, we offer no means for calculating this content, although it would seem that, in such simple cases as those just mentioned, we might be able to decide whether one statement contains more information than another. An utterance that can alter a hearer's state of knowledge in several particulars would seem to contain more information than one that accomplishes less.

It is important, however, that we distinguish between information content and other features of a message, such as its utility or truth value, with which information content is apt to be confused. We would argue that the usefulness to an individual of some particular information is a feature that depends upon circumstances external to the process of communication, and has nothing to do with information. The statement "There will be a deep frost tonight in Tulare County" describes a predicted future state of affairs in a particular locality. The final effect of this utterance will depend upon whether the hearer is a citrus grower in Tulare County, a citrus grower in Florida, an orthopedic surgeon in Tulare County, or a cable car operator in San Francisco. The response of a hearer to this news may depend upon the particular schemata available, as David Rumelhart [102] has suggested, which provide a frame of reference for its interpretation. Yet the statement itself, if it is understood, will first change the knowledge states of these hearers in a similar way. The implications and consequences of the statement will be different for each, but their personal knowledge of the world will initially be changed in generally similar ways. Unless we can distinguish between features that are intrinsic to "information" and those that are not, a theory of information consisting of anything less than a complete theory of human behavior appears unlikely.

The value or utility of information can be estimated in economic, political, or aesthetic terms, and this may be the sole reason for its being sought or given. But such measures of information depend upon the particularity of situations, which frustrates any attempt at formal measurement. We propose, therefore, that information content is to be measured in terms of what an utterance or sentence contains that could change a listener's or reader's knowledge state.

Consider these two sentences:

The king suffered a heart attack while playing golf with Mr. X, and died immediately.

Mr. X suffered a heart attack while playing golf with the king, and died immediately.

The sentences appear to be completely symmetrical, and to contain the same amounts of information. The utility or newsworthiness or surprise value of these sentences may be quite different, however, depending upon circumstances that are external to the sentences but specific to the context, for example, the king of what? (the King of Jazz?), whether the king was young or old, or whether Mr. X was the king's golf instructor or the president of France.

It is also necessary to distinguish between the information content of a statement and its truth content. Consider the statements "Jupiter is larger than Venus," and "Venus is larger than Jupiter." Each of these sentences makes an assertion about a state of affairs which, if understood, would invoke changes of equal extent in the knowledge state of a person who was ignorant of the subject matter. They would appear to have equal information contents, although their truth contents differ sharply. For obvious reasons, we place a high value on truth; the simple fact is that truth is more useful to us than error. In practice, knowing the true state of affairs can have, in fact, a considerable "survival" value. We are sometimes able to distinguish between the information content of a message and its truth content and, in general, it is worth making the effort. For our purposes, however, we will adopt the viewpoint of Zelig Harris that ". . . language is a structure for indicating (indeed, for transmitting) information; it does not have any basic equipment . . . for distinguishing truth" [56].

2.4 An Information Model

The "things" about which utterances, written sentences, or road signs are concerned we will call *nominals* since most of these things have names, and all are nameable.[3] The properties we can attribute to these nominals we will call *attributes*. In sentences of natural language, these would be referred to as the subjects and predicates, respectively, but we will adopt our more neutral terminology in order to deal with nonlinguistic communication processes as well. We will represent the nominals by N, and the attributes by A, so that the utterance "grass is green" would be represented by the forms:

$$(N \parallel A) \text{ or (grass } \parallel \text{ green)}$$

with the nominal and attribute being separated by double vertical strokes, denoting "having the attribute(s)," and the whole included in parentheses. We will call this expression an *information statement,* and require of it that it meet the completeness condition. The information statement is thus analogous to a sentence in natural language.[4]

Most of the information processes with which we will be engaged involve the declarative form. We sacrifice no generality thereby since it is a matter of ordinary experience that "Questions may be asked by uttering declarative sentences, commands may be issued by uttering interrogatory sentences, and so on. We may therefore distinguish between the grammatical structure of a sentence and the kind of communicative act that is performed...." [74].

Consider these sentences:

"Where is the post office?"

"I do not know where the post office is."

"Tell me how to find the post office."

All these sentences call upon a hearer for the same response, though grammatically they are, respectively, a question, a declaration, and a command.

Spoken language is called upon to perform a variety of functions that are not required of written language, and it is necessarily a different form of communication. Conversations follow social protocols, which are a part of the communicative convention rather than a part of the language; one may pause to allow a hearer to interrupt, or one may not, depending upon the circumstances. We may say something softly, stridently, hurriedly, or anxiously. Grammar has nothing to do with this. Spoken language also has tools that may be used for the sole purpose of ensuring that the communication channel is open—"Do you understand me?" "Pay attention!" and the like. We do not have these tools in the written language, and must employ other means. We realize sometimes (perhaps to our regret) that we can speak more rapidly than we can think, but we know that we can think faster than we can write. When we attempt to communicate very rapidly, we may press language to its limits. Lotfi Zadeh has put it this way: "...the pressure for brevity of discourse tends to make natural language *maximally ambiguous* in the sense that the level of ambiguity in human communication is usually near the limit of what is disambiguable through the use of an external body of knowledge which is shared by the parties in discourse" [143]. As we shall see later, natural language may be ambiguous for other reasons, as well.

The completeness condition requires that we have at least one N and one A, and our notation must reflect this. The utterance "grass is green" is of the form $(N \parallel A)$, and is complete. The utterances "grass" or "green" would have either the form $(N \parallel -)$ or $(- \parallel A)$, we cannot tell which. These forms are also incomplete and, when standing alone, they do not convey information.[5] A lengthier and information-rich utterance like "Oak leaves, grass, shrubbery, . . . are eaten by cows, deer, goats, . . ." would be represented in the form $(N_1, N_2, N_3, \ldots \parallel A_1, A_2, A_3, \ldots)$. There is no limit to how many Ns or As could be included, except for matters of economy and clarity. Ordinary utterances and sentences are created in order to attain certain purposes, and their lengths and constructions are dictated by these purposes, not by the rules of grammar.

It is necessary to introduce another convention into our notation. In describing actual objects or in communicating generally, we always leave many things unsaid. These unstated attributes may remain so for a number of reasons. Most commonly it is because they would not serve our communicative purpose to mention them. I may have reason to speak of my dog—"Lance is in the living room with muddy feet"—which would be represented as

$(N \parallel A_1, A_2, \ldots)$. The ellipses after the As remind me that other attributes could be attributed to Lance as well—that he is hungry or that he is seven years old—but these would be irrelevant to the purpose of my utterance. Attributes are also omitted for other reasons, or we may have no knowledge of them, either because we have not troubled to make the necessary observations, or because we have found it impossible to do so. We may, at first, describe a patient as appearing flushed, anxious, and breathing rapidly:

$$(N \parallel A_1, A_2, A_3, \ldots) \tag{1}$$

and then, after a physical examination, add that he is also feverish, has a rapid pulse, and basilar rales.[6]

$$(N \parallel A_1, A_2, A_3, A_4, A_5, A_6, \ldots) \tag{2}$$

We would then continue the observation of the patient, perhaps obtaining sputum cultures and a chest X-ray, but we would never order *all* the tests that are available, nor would we ever be able to find out everything we might wish to know. We shall consider the information statements (1) and (2) as being in the *open*[7] form, recognizing explicitly the existence of additional though unstated attributes.

An information statement may also have unstated or potential nominals. These, however, are of a different character, and are used when we wish to draw attention to the existence of unstated objects that share the same properties. Although it is true (under certain circumstances) that "grass is green":

$$(N \parallel A_1, \ldots) \tag{3}$$

it may be useful to be able to go beyond this, and assert that "frogs and grass are green":

$$(N_1, N_2, \ldots \parallel A_1, \ldots) \tag{4}$$

By placing the ellipses after the nominals, we indicate explicitly that there are other green things. Having once taken this step, we must be careful about including other attributes, such as that frogs have four legs, and attempting to add this fact to the statement.

This, of course, we could not do. Or, to use a medical example, we can properly write:

$$(\text{pneumonia, encephalitis, hepatitis}, \ldots \parallel \text{fever}, \ldots) \qquad (5)$$

indicating that these diseases all have fever as an attribute. This seems correct enough but, if we should recall that a particular feverish patient had pleuritic pain, rales, and increased sputum production, and we wished to modify (5) to reflect this, we could only write:

$$(\text{pneumonia} \parallel \text{fever, pleuritic pain, rales, increased sputum}, \ldots)$$
$$(6)$$

since the newly added attributes are those of neither encephalitis nor hepatitis. As we shall see later when we consider the diagnostic process, one of the common strategies is to "rule out" certain possibilities through further observation. It is our medical knowledge, combined with clinical observations, that enables us to create information statements, as shown in (5), and then to transform them, as shown in (6).

The differences in purpose reflected by (5) and (6) (a process vital to diagnosis) introduces an important issue concerning the ways we think about and describe the world. Statement (5) draws attention to a number of things, all of which share a single stated property. Because of our desire to introduce order into our perception of the world, we actively seek out such generalizations in order to bring many members into a single class or family of things (in this case, febrile diseases). This tendency expresses itself in our search for universals, and underlies our impulse to look for uniformity in nature. When such unifying concepts as Newtonian mechanics or relativity are created, they provide us with great power and insight. Yet such powerful generalizations are found rarely, and we must frequently deal with single and unconnected things. Our descriptions then become particular, as illustrated in (6). By limiting our attention to some single thing, however, we may say a great deal about it. In order to extend the attributes in (6), we need only add something more about pneumonia, but to add attributes to (5) requires that we have knowledge of a larger portion of the world.

Having introduced the concept of open information statements, the reader may well ask whether there are any that are "closed." There are indeed. If we are given a circle C, with radius r, and center at point x, y, we might begin by writing:

$$(C \parallel r, x, y, \dots) \tag{7}$$

But what more could then be said about C which would warrant our using the open form? The answer, of course, is nothing. Instead we must write:

$$(C \parallel r, x, y) \tag{8}$$

indicating that C has no further attributes. It is not the case that C may have properties which we were too lazy to record, or that at some future time mathematicians might discover additional features about C which are presently unknown. The circle C is simply defined as the (infinite) set of points lying in a plane at a distance r from point x, y.[8] Axiomatic systems such as mathematics do not permit the further attribution of features that are not deducible from the axioms themselves, and in this important sense they form closed systems. Circles, in Euclidean geometry, cannot have color, nor can lines have thickness. We cannot go on and freely assert such properties. Instead, we are constrained by the Euclidean axioms.

Closed systems such as these (including axiomatic systems and formal games) need not be regarded as simple because of this. Many are enormously complicated. We cannot predict the future discoveries that may be made in mathematics or in rule-governed games. We do not know the prime numbers that remain to be discovered, nor can we say anything about the chess positions that remain unanalyzed. But, from our knowledge of the rules governing these activities, we can eliminate the possibility of certain kinds of surprises. We can be assured that someone will not discover a new prime number that is even, or that a rook will suddenly attack on a diagonal. The rules forbid such things. With open systems and, especially, with ordinary objects in the natural world (where we know some, but never all, of the rules), we can have no guarantee against surprises. The known laws of nature may provide evidence against certain kinds of results, yet major discoveries in science are always surprises. And we have no basis for expecting that these kinds of surprises will not continue to occur. Since we are concerned primarily with natural objects in medicine, the open form of the information statement will nearly always be the appropriate one.

Since this information model has necessarily been introduced through the use of examples expressed in natural language (ordinary written words and sentences), there is some risk that this might be taken as an attempt to model language. That is not our intent. We will use this model in an attempt to illustrate certain properties of descriptive statements, but this effort should not be taken as an attempt to explain how language functions. Information and language are different kinds of things and, while the transfer of information may be the primary purpose of natural language, there are other means to this end. The lecturer, the cartoonist, the mime, and the mapmaker may all share a similar purpose, and it is not our aim here to explore the grammars of the different "languages" they employ.

2.5 Fact Statements About the World

It is obvious enough, when we reflect upon it, that our descriptions of natural objects do not just happen to be incomplete, they are *necessarily* incomplete. Yet even incomplete descriptions may be overly detailed and burdensome, and do not serve us well. Useful information permits us to do something: to understand a phenomenon, or to choose between courses of action. In all our communications we say less than what could be said in the effort to say what it is necessary to say. One of the ways we have of supplying this emphasis is by *abstraction*. We may do this consciously when we attempt to summarize a long piece of writing in a shorter one. We accomplish this by limiting ourselves to topics we believe to be essential. But we perform abstractions unconsciously all the time—we certainly did when we were writing the original piece. Every description of a natural object, process, or state of affairs is an abstraction for the simple reasons that we can never know everything there is to know, nor say all that might be said.

Intrinsic to the process of abstraction is the ability of an observer to distinguish between what is relevant in a particular context and what is merely adventitious. How we go about this is far from clear. Karl Popper (among others) emphasizes that we have a certain set of expectations regarding objects or processes which guides our observation [100]. He points out that observation is "theory laden," that we pay more attention to certain features of a state of affairs because we have a theory that ascribes a greater pertinence to them, or in which they are believed to play a more significant role. If we are able to distinguish the relevant from the irrelevant in observation, no matter how we succeed in accomplishing this, we can also do it in describing our observations. We may describe a patient as lying in bed propped up on three pillows, with an ashen complexion, struggling for breath, and having distended neck veins. But in a medical context we would not add that the patient was dressed in blue pajamas or wore sideburns. These and a host of other attributes would be ignored as we form the clinical abstraction of a patient for the purpose of discussing the case with another physician, or for writing a case report.

2.6 The Matter of Questions

Spoken questions, and dialogue generally, might appear to violate the completeness criterion we have proposed. Speech, unlike formal written communication, is often carelessly constructed. When we talk, we rush on pell-mell, restrained only by our hearer's comprehension. In a conversation, much of the information is transferred by phrases and single words (and by gestures and "body language," as well) rather than by grammatically complete sentences. That understanding is possible at all emphasizes the critical role played by context. The significance of context always seems to be underestimated because much of it derives from the situation in which a speaker and hearer find themselves, and it is implicit rather than explicit. Although complete sentences have their own meanings, there is always additional meaning to be found in a collection of them (e.g., a paragraph) that cannot be localized to any particular sentence. Consider the effects of rearranging the sentences of a novel. The formal meaning of the individual sentences would be largely unaffected by this, but the context would be destroyed and many sentences would become incomprehensible. The notion of a context, or a "train of thought," is something beyond the grasp of grammar. Conversations are borne along by a focus on a topic, and by an interest shared by speakers and hearers in particular subjects, and fragmentary utterances involving references to things embedded in the context rather than being explicit in the conversation are perfectly understandable.

The structure of questions displays a number of interesting features. One of these is that, while they request information, they *must also provide information*. Questions must do this (i.e., satisfy the completeness requirement) if they are themselves to be understood. Moreover, questions must explain, with some exactness, the nature of the information requested. The question "Who is the tall man in the tweed suit standing behind you?" informs the hearer of at least half a dozen different things, and also states what is desired. This question can be acted upon, whereas the question "Who is that man?" cannot be acted upon in the absence of other clues. Questions tend to have a reciprocal relation with their appropriate responses. A question that seeks highly specific information will necessarily contain a great deal of information if its purpose is to be achieved. The reply to such a question may frequently be brief.

"Is there a mailbox on the northeast corner of the intersection of Post and Taylor streets in San Francisco?" "No." ("Yes.")

Questions that contain too few, or include irrelevant, attributes may fail in specifying what is desired. They would be taken as vague and, unless remedied, could only prompt equally vague answers. We shall see later that in questioning patients, retrieving documents, or searching computerized data bases, the creation of suitable questions may be a complex process. Question formation is no less difficult or important than the creation of satisfactory descriptions. Indeed, when someone shows particularly keen insight into a problem, we often remark that he or she "has asked the right questions."

2.7 Understanding Communications

Understanding a communication means that in some way we have made cognitive contact with the creator of the message. A dog's scratching at the back door in order to be let out has its intention realized when we open the door. Before we are moved to do this, we must first understand the message. If an interactive computer program indicates to us that particular data are to be entered, our response in properly doing so satisfies some programmer's desire, even though this may have been originally expressed years before and miles away. Human communications succeed when a declaration, an expectation, or an intention formed in one mind is apprehended by another and acknowledged. Whether or not an attempted communication succeeds depends upon a number of factors. We shall examine here those that seem to be of the most importance to us.

Since human communications succeed most of the time, and because they are influenced by unknown subconscious mechanisms, it is easy to overlook the necessary conditions that are involved. Before we can say anything at all we must first isolate some particular thing out of the universe of possible things to speak about. Ordinarily, we do much more than this. Though our single sentences or utterances may deal with isolated and distinct things, our short-term collections of them will tend to deal with groups of related things. Our utterances or writings will, in short, have topics. Once a hearer's or reader's attention has been drawn to a particular subject matter, it is usual for the next utterance or sentence to refer to the same topic or to a closely related one. Conversations and discussions construct contexts. That is why we preface major shifts in the thrust of a conversation with such signals as "To change the subject..." or "By the way..."

The use of topics is a common source of context. If one were talking about an election, a footrace, or a tennis match, the statement "Jones will probably beat Smith" would not be misunderstood as implying that Jones was likely to assault Smith. The context allows us to disambiguate such competing meanings, and to achieve understanding. But topics cannot provide the sole source of context. If they did, we could never begin a conversation nor could we follow the transitions between unrelated topics.

Although we instinctively recognize when a statement or utterance is out of context, we have no formal rules for deciding the matter. That is, we have no automatic means for determining at the moment of hearing whether a statement is relevant or not. If we hear the utterance "Consider the lilies of the field..." we have no basis for judging its relevance until we hear what follows. Written and spoken communications are sequential in time, and relevance is hostage to the future. Something that may appear irrelevant at a given moment may later be connected up or justified.

Through custom or courtesy, a speaker's utterance may be taken to be relevant, but, if we are kept waiting too long for our expectation to be fulfilled, we quickly lose interest.

It is difficult to imagine encounters between humans, no matter how exaggerated the example, which would be completely free of context since they occur in shared situations. The only instance of a completely context-free encounter would seem to be that of "communicating" with a computer. In this case there can be no context, beyond that which is expressed in the programs. Since in human communication a context is essential for the resolution of ambiguity, the absence of context might seem to be a fatal obstacle in attempting to communicate with computers. It turns out that by far the easiest way to avoid ambiguity when using computers is not by attempting to supply the computer program with a sufficiently rich context (this being, in general, an unsolved problem) but by a direct resolution of ambiguity itself. This resolution is accomplished by the use of ambiguity-free languages and this, of course, is what computer languages are for.

Humans do it the other way around, and use language that is rich, ambiguous, fuzzy, and imprecise, but they succeed in making themselves understood through the use of context.[9] Natural language has evolved in response to the need of humans to talk about a great variety of things. Computer languages, in contrast, are designed to interface with the small set of primitive, logical operations that computers are engineered to carry out. The limited extent to which such languages can be used to describe the ordinary world will be considered later. Having a suitable context, then, is necessary for the understanding of a message, and this may either be provided by the message itself or lie external to it. There are other requirements, as well.

A message that satisfies the syntactic rules of a language has passed only a first test. A second requirement is that the appropriate words must be chosen for particular objects. That is, the words selected must succeed in capturing the speaker's intended meaning. Chomsky's well-known sentence, "Colorless green ideas sleep furiously," has been argued to be syntactically correct. The reason it cannot be understood is because of its disregard of semantics and, because of this, the sentence is regarded as meaningless. How such results can come about accidentally—rather than purposely, as in this example—will be seen in the next chapter.

To ensure understanding, a message must pass yet another test, one that linguists include under the subject of pragmatics. That is, a successful message must refer to some comprehensible state of affairs. The statement "*A* is greater than *B* and is less than *B*" is syntactically and semantically satisfactory, but we cannot understand it except, perhaps, metaphorically. The reason for this is that it corresponds to no state of affairs in the world that we have experienced or can experience. Understandable statements about the world correspond to the world in a particular way, and messages that do not accomplish this cannot be understood. That a message must correspond in some way to the structure and the rules of the world is a further requirement for its being understood. Robert Schank has written:

> ... suppose *Paris Match* had every word in French changed into English, but no syntactical rearrangement was done. It would be comprehensible. The rules of French grammar are not crucial in understanding French, but the rules of the world are. [108]

I believe that Schank seriously overstates his case here. Grammar is not all that dispensable, and an error in tense or mood can readily lead to the failure to understand a proposition. But his point is well-intentioned; a statement that defies the rules of the world invites misunderstanding.

Finally, the "information" and "facts" that we are considering are not things that are just lying about out there in the world, independent of people and of minds. Descriptions of facts, and information, are the creations of humans with minds. But for humans to be able to describe facts and produce information there must be a world out there. Because of the importance of the world to our descriptions of it, we must now examine the relations between them.

3

The Structure of Descriptions

3.1 Structural Features of the World

The study and practice of medicine involve dealing with a diverse collection of natural and artificial objects. The language of medicine, dealing as it does with living things like men and microbes, natural ones like vitamins and digitalis, and artificial things like pacemakers, comes into contact with many different aspects of the world. It will be our aim here to consider how our observations of the world, and our descriptions of the things we study, are influenced by structural features of the world. In particular, we will be interested in our descriptions of living things, to see in what ways these may differ from our descriptions of other objects.

The evolution of our minds has occurred in close relation to the world around us; our minds expect to find a world at the other end of our perceptual channels. In experiments on sensory deprivation, for example [58], one can place a diving helmet on a subject, immerse him in warm water, in the darkness and in silence, and the experimental subject typically falls asleep. Upon awakening, he finds himself disoriented, and hallucinations may occur. Minds seem to need (or expect) the world for confirmation of continuity and if, under experimental conditions such as these, we do not perceive a world "out there," it appears that we create one (hallucinate). We also expect the world to have a degree of permanence, to appear in the same general form as it has in our past experience. Many optical illusions are designed to trick the mind by utilizing this expectation. A photograph of a well-known public figure, if viewed upside down, will usually not be recognized. We do not expect to see humans in that orientation, and our mechanisms for the recognition of faces fails us under those circumstances.

The realization that the natural world could be observed, described, and analyzed by various observers with generally consistent results seems to have come as a substantial discontinuity in the development of Western thought. This event has been referred to as the "discovery of nature," and as the "introduction of rational criticism and debate." It has been spoken of as the "Greek miracle" [72]. This idea that the world is both susceptible to study and worthy of it seems to have become popular first with Thales and the Milesian school of philosopher-scientists. The importance of this development has been described by Anaxagoras: "All things were in chaos when Mind arose and made order" [53]. Only when it was appreciated that there was order in nature did science become possible.

Although, as we have noted, the greater part of our knowledge of the world is acquired by direct experience ("knowledge by acquaintance") it is knowledge of the second kind ("knowledge by description") that makes possible the organized and cooperative activities of science and education. Knowledge by description makes possible the miracle of knowing something we have never experienced ourselves. This process of converting knowledge of the first type into the second, of being able to articulate our experiential (acquaintance) knowledge, is fundamental to its verification. How then do we create these descriptions of the world?

We shall begin by examining what it is that we can say about ordinary matter. Observations of many different kinds support the theory that matter is composed of particles known as protons, neutrons, and electrons, and that each of these objects has certain characteristic properties: mass, electric charge, and magnetic moment.[1] It is only by means of these properties that these objects can be distinguished. This particular theory further asserts that these particles have no internal structure, and that the three attributes, or observables, are all that can be known about them. Protons are thus characterized by their (rest) mass (m_p), their electric charge (q_p), and their magnetic moment (μ_p). All objects that are found to have just these attributes belong to the class labeled "proton." We will therefore write:

$$(\text{Proton} \parallel m_\text{p}, q_\text{p}, \mu_\text{p}, \ldots) \tag{1}$$

This statement can be taken as having either of two interpretations: (a) if, on one hand, we encounter an object having mass m_p, electric charge q_p, and magnetic moment μ_p, we are obliged (under this theory) to call this object a proton. If, on the other hand (b), we know what protons are, and we are then told that something is a proton, we would expect to find it to have just the attributes, m_p, q_p, and μ_p. The process (a) works from right to left, and is related to such cognitive processes as *naming* or *recognizing*. Having been provided with the attributes, the information statement then tells us that the appropriate name is "proton." Or if we were already familiar with the name and we found ourselves confronted with these attributes, we would recognize their co-occurrence and the name "proton" would come to mind. The process (b) works from left to right, and it is associated with such notions as *explaining,* or *describing.* If someone wants to know what a proton is, all we can do is to provide this list of attributes and then, if necessary, explain the attributes. It is of interest to note that, whereas (1) implies only two processes (being given the *A*'s, which then point to the *N,* or being presented with an *N,* which will call up a particular set of *A*'s), a number of different terms are commonly used in speaking of these cognitive processes. Our information model—the ($N \parallel A$) model—suggests that, although there may be only a relatively few primitive information processes, we may employ them for a number of different reasons and that when we do so they take on different names.

We shall call the attributes we have listed in (1) *necessary attributes* since, to be entitled to membership in the class "proton," and to bear this name, an object must have precisely these attributes. It is also the case with these particular objects (protons) that some of their attributes are also *sufficient* for class membership.[2] But there are a great many protons in the universe, bound or free, having various locations and velocities. If we are to speak about a particular proton, we need a means for distinguishing it from all other protons. It is important for us to be able to single out a particular member of a class. We can do this in the case of material objects by means of spatio-temporal references. If we wish to refer to the proton that caused *this particular* cloud chamber track, we can list its successive positions at different times and, in effect, say *this one.* We can also determine its other attributes, such as velocity or energy. We shall call attributes such as position, velocity, and energy *contingent attributes.* They play no role in defining membership in a class or in naming, but they serve to particularize an object within a class or to provide us with more information about a given thing. For elementary particles (or, as we shall see, for *simple* objects generally), the number of necessary attributes are few, and they are readily distinguished from contingent attributes. When we come later to consider more complex objects (in particular the tangible objects of everyday experience, and the things we speak of in medicine), we will find that their attributes become vastly more numerous, and the objects themselves are less readily subject to precise definition. We will also find that with complex objects it is no longer a simple matter to distinguish between their necessary and contingent attributes. This will have important consequences when we attempt to classify "things," such as living organisms, or biological phenomena, such as diseases.

3.2 Hierarchical Structures and the Organization of Matter

The means at our disposal for describing protons are equally applicable to neutrons and electrons, so that we can write in a similar manner:

$$(\text{Neutron} \quad m_n, q_n, \mu_n, \dots), \ (\text{Electron} \quad m_e, q_e, \mu_e, \dots) \qquad (2)$$
(Where the m's, q's, and μ's are those of the designated particles.)

And these objects, too, may be particularized, and referred to individually by using contingent attributes.

Under the same theory of physics, we shall now consider the process of bringing a proton and an electron together to form an entirely new object. Well-known physical principles tell us that, since these particles have opposite electrical charges, they will attract one another. Experiments show that when this occurs a stable object is formed and, in this case, the object formed is known as a hydrogen atom. We can describe this in terms of its constituent particles:

$$(\text{H-atom} \parallel \text{Proton, Electron}, \dots) \qquad (3)$$

It turns out, however, that when hydrogen atoms are observed carefully, still other attributes are to be found. There is more that needs to be said about hydrogen atoms than merely that they consist of a proton and an electron. One of these additional properties is that of *excitation* (excited states): the fact that the hydrogen (or any) atom exists at any given instant in one of a number of permitted energy states, and that it can absorb or emit energy only in amounts corresponding to the energy differences between these states. In order to describe a hydrogen atom more completely, we must include this property as well.

(Level 2) (H-atom ‖ Proton, Electron, excited states, . . .)   (4)

(Level 1) (Proton ‖ m_p, q_p, μ_p, . . .) (Electron ‖ m_e, q_e, μ_e, . . .)

We can then write the information statements for the proton and electron immediately below that of the hydrogen atom, and indicate the relations between them. These linked information statements of (4) stand, respectively, as descriptions of the hydrogen atom, and of the proton and electron. We note that we now have two different levels of description: one suitable for atoms (level 2), and another for the subatomic particles (level 1). By arranging these descriptions in this form, we can indicate the hierarchical relations that derive from their part-whole relationship.

When we speak of a hydrogen atom, it is the nominal, the "thing," to which our listener's attention is drawn. The hydrogen atom's having (consisting of) a proton and an electron, and being capable of excitation are attributes that can be asserted of it. And, again, with the proton, our description of *it* nominalizes it, and we can list its attributes. In doing this, our description now occurs at a lower level. Something, it would appear, *cannot be both a nominal and an attribute at the same descriptive level* when we deal with hierarchical systems.

We have considered Whitehead's claim about thought being necessarily concerned with "things." To this we must now add the corollary that attention confers "thinghood." When we are thinking about some particular thing, and that object occupies our attention, our focusing of attention establishes the descriptive level. To get rid of the classical idea of universal "substance,"

Russell pointed out that a "thing" can only be conceived of as "a bundle of qualities" [103]. Our model of an information statement exemplifies this.

One feature of (4) requires further comment. From where does the attribute excitation arise? We cannot trace its origin to the next lower level, as we can for the proton and electron. It is something that does not exist at level 1. Free protons and electrons cannot (as a matter of physics) have this attribute. Furthermore, there seems to be nothing in any theory sufficient to account for matters at level 1 that would predict such a property.[3] The attribute excitation, which occurs and can be observed at level 2, simply has no meaning at level 1. There is no referent occupying the lower level for the word *excitation*.

Such a property is spoken of as an *emergent* property. Peter Medawar has described emergence in this way:

> In hierarchically organized systems, especially in biology, the appearance at some tier of the hierarchy of a novelty which is not obviously predictable or foreseeable in terms of anything that has preceded it. Thus consciousness or cerebration has been said to have "emerged" in the evolution of higher primates. Much earnest and confused thought surrounds the notion that emergence is a kind of evolutionary strategem which explains the appearance of novelties. [79]

As can be seen in our example, however, the process of emergence is by no means limited to biology or to the higher hierarchical levels but occurs already at the lowest levels in our descriptions of matter. Neither, would it appear, does the phenomenon of emergence have any particular explanatory power. On the contrary, it seems to call for an explanation rather than providing one.

We shall now proceed to consider the next higher structural level of matter, and its description. If we bring together two hydrogen atoms and an oxygen atom (under suitable conditions), we can form a water molecule:

(Level 3) (Water molecule ‖ Hydrogen atom$_1$,   (5)
             Hydrogen atom$_2$, Oxygen atom, . . .
             covalent bonds, vibrational states, electric dipole
             moment, . . .)

A description of a water molecule must include its constituents and its properties. The newly emergent properties of *covalent bonds, vibrational states,* and *electric dipole moment,* which we find in a water molecule, are again properties that do not occur with isolated atoms. There are others as well, and the higher we proceed in the hierarchical organization of matter, the more numerous the emergent properties become with each additional descriptive level.

In addition to the emergent attributes that appear at successively higher levels, another feature sets in, which further affects the process of naming—that of *individuality.* This evolves from the fact that higher-level objects possess more "degrees of freedom." This expression derives from the increased number of coordinates required for the physical description of systems consisting of multiple unconstrained objects, such as the molecules of a gas. But it is also an apt description for the tension that occurs in nature between *uniformity* and *novelty.* Low-level objects, such as protons and electrons, appear monotonously alike. When we turn to higher-level objects, such as dogs, we find that they share characteristics (necessary attributes) that permit us to assign them to this class (dogs) but, in addition, we see that each member of the class displays a multitude of individual and novel features enabling us to recognize readily a particular breed as unique. When such clearly distinguishable objects are referred to by the same name, the naming process becomes ambiguous. This characteristic, as with the appearance of emergent properties, does not arise suddenly at any particular hierarchical level, but increases steadily as successively higher levels are examined. This appearance of uniqueness has an important effect on the processes of naming and of class assignment. And as with emergence, its onset is most clearly seen at the lower levels.

When we use the word *proton,* we denote a class of objects that are all alike. At this level, something approaching Plato's universals might seem close at hand. When we move up to the next level, at which the descriptions of atoms lie, we might imagine constructing atoms by sticking together various combinations of protons, neutrons, and electrons. If we were to attempt this, we would find that not all of these imagined collections exist as permanent objects in the world. There is, for example, no object consisting of two neutrons and an electron and, even if we were to succeed experimentally in bringing three such particles together momentarily, the collection would have no permanence. We do, however, find stable objects consisting of a proton and an electron; a proton, a neutron, and an electron; and a proton, two neutrons, and an electron. The rules of nature permit the formation of these three objects, all share the properties of having a nuclear charge of unity, a single valence electron, and of being stable. These shared properties also happen to be those that are important for chemical behavior, and the class of objects having these properties are known, in chemical language, as hydrogen atoms. Although alike chemically, these objects can be readily distinguished from one another so that in the language of atomic physics they are known as hydrogen, deuterium, and tritium, respectively.

Even at this low level in the organization of matter, we are confronted with a problem in the proper choice of a name (or word) for an object. We regard this as a problem because we like to suppose that words and objects fall into a tidy one-to-one correspondence, and that if we choose a word carefully enough we can always point to a particular thing without ambiguity. But we will discover, as we did with emergence, that when we attempt to describe natural objects, ambiguity and fuzziness make their appearance at very low levels. In dealing with higher-level objects, particularly the common ones met with in everyday activities, ambiguity is not an unfortunate by-product of complexity, but a powerful feature, which makes it possible for us to deal with it. It is an old observation that practical human communications would be impossible without the use of ambiguity.

Instead of continuing this building process in detail, level by level, we will sketch, in figure 3.1, some of the general hierarchical features of matter. The diagram rapidly becomes too cumbersome to show all the linkages between levels, and the level-numbering system has been changed to indicate that the diagram can be further extended down as well as up. Elementary particle physics is already providing us with well-organized descriptive levels below that of protons and electrons.

Examining the figure more closely, we will note the following systematic features:

1. As we shift our attention up one level, nominals become attributes; this we will refer to as the $N \rightarrow A$ shift ($\rightarrow$ = "becomes").

2. The attributes that exist at a particular level disappear as we move up one level, and become *embedded*.

3. Emergent attributes come into existence with each increase of level, and contribute to the behavior of objects at the level of emergence and at all levels above, although they subsequently become embedded. A property emerging at a lower level, such as atomic excitation, may participate in a process that itself only emerges at a still higher level; metabolism is an example.

4. Not representable in the figure is the increase in the ambiguity of reference from word to object(s), the growth of fuzziness, the disappearance of uniformity, the rise of individuality, and an increased difficulty in distinguishing necessary from contingent attributes.

When we proceed downward, these changes are reversed:

1. Aspects become nominalized: the A ➤ N shift.

2. Previously embedded properties become *disclosed*.

3. Emergent properties disappear at the level immediately below that at which they emerged.

4. Word reference becomes less ambiguous as the referents become both fewer and sharper, fuzziness is reduced, individuality is replaced by uniformity, and necessity and contingency are more readily distinguished.[4]

When we deal with natural objects such as hydrogen atoms or water molecules, which are themselves formed of constituent objects, a descriptive level higher than what suffices for the description of their components becomes necessary if our knowledge of them is to be adequately represented. It is thus not by mere whim that we create a molecular level of description when we attempt to describe the state of affairs that occurs when atoms become bonded together. A new molecular vocabulary is required in order to talk about such emergent properties as "vibrational and rotational states," "optical activity," "electric dipole moment," and the like. These terms have no referents at the atomic level, and the vocabulary sufficient for atoms is inadequate for the description of molecules. As we examine objects still higher in the hierarchy, new properties continue to emerge and still higher-level languages are required.

Although we began our considerations at the bottom of the hierarchy of material objects (the "classical" elementary particles), we social, economic, political structures

+2	(tribe $\parallel$ family$_1$, family$_2$, ... *social rules*, ...)
+1	(family $\parallel$ father, mother, children, ... *customs*, ...)
level 0	(man $\parallel$ animal, ... *highly developed consciousness, complex language, complex tools*, ...)
−1	(animal $\parallel$ skeleton, organ$_1$, ... muscle, ... *integument*, ... *complex behavior*, ...)
−2	(organ/tissue $\parallel$ cell$_1$, cell$_2$, ... *connective tissue*, ...)
−3	(cell $\parallel$ nucleus, organelle$_1$, ... *reproduction*, ...)
−4	(organelle $\parallel$ membrane, ... *ordered chemical synthesis* ... *compartmentation*, ...)
−5	(membrane $\parallel$ structural protein$_1$, enzyme$_1$, ... *lipid layers*, ... *permeability*, ... *enzyme arrangement*, ...)
−6	(protein $\parallel$ tyrosine, alanine, ... *tertiary structure*, ...)
−7	(amino acid $\parallel$ H-atom$_1$, 0-atom$_1$, ... *vibrational states*, ... *covalent bonds*, ...)
−8	(H-atom $\parallel$ proton, electron, ... *excited states*, ... *ionization potential*, ...)
−9	(proton $\parallel$ mass$_p$, charge$_p$, magnetic moment$_p$, ...)

quarks, elementary particles

Figure 3.1. The descriptions of natural objects can be expressed in (N $\parallel$ A) form and allocated to appropriate hierarchical levels to produce a knowledge network.

could just as well have started at some arbitrarily higher one and worked our way down. Historically, our knowledge of nature has been acquired in just this way. Essays on the philosophy of mind commonly begin such a discussion as this with the everyday tangible objects that we experience directly. If we had followed this top-down course, we would have found the language appropriate at one descriptive level to be excessively rich at the next lower one. Since it contained terms corresponding to newly emergent properties, these terms would have no referents at the lower level. But we would also have needed new terms for the embedded properties that were disclosed as we proceeded downward.

The descriptive levels of figure 3.1 should not be thought of as a rigid ladder on which all the rungs stand out with equal sharpness. Our attention cannot span such breadth and take in detail at the same time. The rung of a ladder with which we may be preoccupied at a particular moment corresponds to the level at which our attention is directed. And we can see clearly only the rungs immediately above and below us. As we shift our attention up or down, some rungs will come into focus as we approach them, and others will disappear as we leave them behind. We know the other rungs are there somewhere, but it is difficult to visualize them until they are fairly close at hand. We cannot have before our mind's eye at the same time the rung for "headache" (which is an attribute of a conscious organism) and the one for "aspirin" (a molecule), although we know full well that we can work our way from one to the other. We must be able to do this if we hope to explain the effect of aspirin upon headache.

We may refer to L_i as the language that has been found to have the necessary richness required to describe a state of affairs at the ith level, and which contains only terms having referents at this level, that is, it is not unnecessarily rich. Such a language then is both necessary and sufficient for the description of the natural world at this level. What happens if this language is employed in an attempt to describe matters at some other level? If the misapplication is downward, one risks creating meaningless sentences such as "What is the color of a water molecule?" or "This action produces pain in the cell membrane." In order to avoid nonsense such as this, our descriptions must consist of words taken from the vocabulary of a single level or from the vocabularies of closely adjacent levels. In transparent examples such as the preceding ones, no great harm is done, yet language misapplication downward can cause considerable mischief. The nonmetaphorical application of human predicates to lower organisms ("my plant seems sad") and the use of predicates appropriate for the description of living things with inanimate objects ("intelligent machines") confuses rather than clarifies. We will examine some of the consequences of such misapplications later.

The use of lower-level languages in describing higher-level objects raises difficulties of a different kind. One is simply that it is a nuisance. It is convenient that we are able to create and use higher-level concepts such as metabolism when we wish to speak about cells or tissues or organisms. This avoids the need for going into such low-level details as excited states, covalent bond opening, electron transport, and oxidation-reductions. It would be extremely awkward to talk about biochemistry using only the language of atomic and molecular physics, but it would be impossible to discuss clinical neurology in this way. It is through the use of high-level or "portmanteau" terms such as *metabolism,* which are packed with multiple meanings, that ordinary conversation becomes possible. If we had to describe our everyday affairs using only lower-level vocabularies, we would have time for little else. Since we would have no terms for dealing with emergent properties, we would be forced to employ lengthy and awkward locutions, and explain these new properties as we went along. How could we begin to speak of things like fear, using only the low-level languages of physics or chemistry? Of course we have never had to attempt this, since things happened the other way around, and natural languages began with the use of words for dealing with everyday objects. Vocabularies for dealing with the very large (planetary systems, galaxies) and the very small (electrons, quarks) were neither needed nor developed until much later.

Implicit in what has been said so far is that our descriptions of natural objects, if they are to be accurate, must in the end reflect the constraints of natural laws.[5] We have not yet referred to the connections between natural laws and our networks of linked sets of information statements. Physical, chemical, and biological laws enter into and determine the relations among attributes, and constrain the way in which nominals may be joined if we are to describe true states of affairs. Because of the hierarchical distance, we cannot speak of forming a chemical bond between a particular carbon atom and a particular elephant, although the carbon atom may well become bonded to another atom that is properly a part of the elephant.

The laws that describe the behavior of elementary particles in isolated atoms continue to describe this behavior when these atoms become parts of biopolymers, tissues, and organs, although by themselves *these laws increasingly fall short of accounting for the behavior of these higher-level objects*. After repeated embedding, the operations of these laws become hidden from us, and their effects may seem in some way to have become attenuated. This impression, however, is the result of our attention being necessarily fixed, at any given moment, upon a particular level. We cannot "see" everything at once, and the presence and effects of embedded attributes can always be disclosed by shifting our attention to lower levels.

To remark that natural laws tend to describe matters at some single level is only to restate the obvious: that atomic physics deals with elementary particles and atoms, that chemistry is concerned with collections of atoms and molecules, and that the laws of biology deal with living organisms. And the atoms comprised in an organism will continue to behave in the ways described by the laws of atomic physics, even though these laws no longer tell the whole story. Low-level laws are necessary but insufficient for the description of the behavior of such high-level things as humans. There are additional laws, entering at successively higher levels (such as the laws of biology and psychology) that are required for the description of the emergent properties.

For sciences like atomic physics, chemistry, and biology to be possible at all, it must be possible to take natural objects apart—not only figuratively but in practice—in order to isolate and study the constituent objects in figure 3.1 in detail. If, upon attempting to dissect a frog, a biologist found that it dissolved into a cloud of elementary particles, he or she would be able to say little about biology or, for that matter, about physiology, anatomy, or molecular biology. But ordinary matter does not behave like that. Everyday objects can be taken apart, layer by layer, and it is this circumstance that justifies our drawing in figure 3.1. These hierarchical levels are not arbitrary structures imposed by us upon nature, but inherent to the way in which natural matter occurs. And these levels represent the only way in which matter can be taken apart, if we are to be left with something to examine. These constituent assemblages are stable and can be studied in detail, and then further taken apart, with the result that we have such fields as chemistry and atomic physics, and the languages that go with them. It is this actual (not conceptual) *decomposability* that is the strongest evidence for the thesis of hierarchical structure of the material world.[6]

3.3 The Nonhierarchical World

The process recounted in the previous section, which leads to the formation of hierarchical structures, should not prompt us to conclude that all the world is so organized. Consider for a moment the formation of such tangible objects as minerals or rocks. We can conceive of a simple assembly process, beginning with, say, single copper atoms, and imagine sticking them together, one at a time, to form a very tiny crystal of copper. At some stage in this building process, the crystal forces will begin to hold the atoms together to form a stable object. At this point, the tiny particle will begin to display properties approaching those of bulk copper. It will take on the crystal form and atomic spacings, display the electrical conductivity, and begin to approach the density of ordinary bulk copper. All these properties are emergent ones, and not one of them is shown by isolated, single copper atoms. But the emergence of these new properties is, in this case, an exceedingly slow one. Unlike the case of hierarchical systems, there is no single step in the assembly process at which these new properties suddenly emerge.

Our collection, in this example, must approach some hundreds or thousands of atoms before it begins to have properties closely resembling those of bulk copper. This behavior is contrasted with the rapid and discontinuous appearance of emergent properties that occurs when *different* kinds of objects are brought together, such as in forming molecules from atoms. Once this copper crystal displays the bulk properties of ordinary copper, the addition of more copper atoms will make no difference—nothing further happens. No new properties arise. Hierarchical systems are not being formed. The aggregation of like objects is not a process rich in the emergence of new properties, nor does ambiguity of reference increase as a result of the sheer increase in size. The phrase "a single crystal of copper'' retains its precise meaning whether we are speaking of a crystal that is a micron in size, or one as large as a loaf of bread.

The crystals of the elements and of their compounds, and mixtures of them including amorphous substances, are the construction materials out of which the nonliving world is built. Thus rocks and mountains and dead planets display a structural poverty compared with living things. For chemical and biological evolution to have occurred at all, there must first have been, it would seem, a fairly thorough, even if local, mixing of matter so that *dissimilar* substances could be brought together in various combinations. It seems plausible that only in this manner could the emergence of novel properties have been favored.

When we speak of the hierarchical and nonhierarchical worlds, and of natural objects and artifacts, we are attempting to classify the world. This has been a preoccupation of philosophers and scientists, beginning with Aristotle, and now includes all professionals. This preoccupation is exemplified by one group of professionals for whom classification is an indispensable activity—the librarians. The proper classification of books and artifacts has long been and still is a subject of paramount importance to them. Although arrangement of books can be wholly arbitrary, for example, with books arranged alphabetically by author, by size, or according to the color of the binding, there are obvious advantages if books and artifacts are categorized or classified to conform to what are referred to as ''natural classes.'' It is convenient if books that deal with the same or related subjects are found gathered together in the same place. The ancient sciences were classified by Aristotle in such a way, and his scheme was employed until the birth of modern science in the Renaissance. The hierarchical classification of the sciences in the supposed order of decreasing generality and increasing complexity (mathematics, astronomy, physics, chemistry, biology, sociology), which was advocated by Auguste Comte in the early nineteenth century, persists today in the Dewey decimal system (and similar schemes) employed by our libraries. This approach, however, exhibits but poorly our modern perception of the structure of the world. Would Comte, for example, still be satisfied with classifying all nonterrestrial matters under ''astronomy''? Not if he had been able to accompany an Apollo mission! In his day, astronomy was largely a matter of applied mathematics and classical mechanics. Today, it includes disciplines as disparate as plasma physics and biology. Yet the influence of the Comtean scheme as a method of classifying the world persists to the present.[7]

That no classification yet developed has been entirely satisfactory is evident from the continuing efforts of librarians and information scientists to devise improved ones. A recent study that considered this problem [69] proposed the following hierarchical scheme:

1. Fundamental particles
2. Nuclei
3. Atoms
4. Molecules
5. Molecular assemblages (natural objects and artifacts)
6. Cells
7. Organisms
8. Human beings
9. Human societies

This modern attempt at classification reflects the structure of the world in a manner not too different from that shown in our figure 3.1, although its allocation of artifacts may appear to some readers as odd. Let us see why.

The levels shown in figure 3.1 represent the relationships among the descriptions of the increasingly complex objects of the non-living natural world and the living world. How then are we to judge the complexity of artifacts? If this were suitably determined, where would their complexity place them with respect to natural objects? The most characteristic thing about an artifact seems to be that it *is* an artifact. Any description of an artifact must begin with this fact. We cannot create an adequate description of such a simple tool as a screwdriver without mentioning that it was made for a particular *human purpose*. If this point were not made, our description would fail to capture the nature of the object. Moreover, it is this feature of artifacts that enables us to recognize them as artifacts and not as objects arising through organic evolution or produced by some chance accident. But when we include such attributes in order to explain the specific human purposes they are intended to serve, we must be prepared to admit still other attributes. A screwdriver would be incomprehensible without the concept of a screw, just as a screw would be incomprehensible without the idea of being able to fasten objects together, and the process of fastening without being able to envision the possibility of constructing other artifacts for still other purposes. To understand the screwdriver, we must know something about these other things as well. Nor can we understand keys without knowing something about locks and doors, not to mention security. Once we acknowledge that such objects are man-made and are created to serve human purposes, their detailed descriptions become enormously complex. Few objects, it might be thought, could be simpler than a copper coin. But in order to describe a coin in a context-free situation requires not only the vocabularies of mining and metallurgy but also of economics and government. The apparent simplicity of common artifacts, which includes most of the objects that surround us in our everyday lives, is quite misleading.

It appears that our descriptions of artifacts must lie at a higher level than level 0 of figure 3.1. Such an allocation seems appropriate because of the historical sequences of evolution, by the increasing complexity of the objects involved, and by our desire to "explain" or account for one thing in terms of others lying at a lower level. Human artifacts must lie at a level higher than that of the human individual, since human purposes are among their attributes. The seeming paradox in assigning "simple" artifacts to a hierarchical level this high stems from the circumstance that our entire lives are spent among such artifacts, and their familiarity is mistaken for simplicity. From the time we arise in the morning, dress, eat, and move on through our daily activities to the time we fall asleep at night, we are immersed in a sea of artificial objects to which, in one form or another, mankind has grown accustomed over thousands of years. It is impossible for us now to recapture the sense of wonder that any one of these artifacts must have occasioned at the time of its discovery or creation. The inventions of weaving and of the button and buttonhole must have been as remarkable in their own times as any of our modern technical achievements.

If this allocation of artifacts is justified, then some of the traditional arguments regarding the relationships of men and machines require reanalysis. So long as machines are regarded as being relatively simple and living things complex (this being sometimes expressed as "the simplest living cell is more complex than the most complicated computer"), it would seem reasonable to attempt to explain an organism in terms of an allegedly simpler machine. We are here using the word *explain* in the sense of accounting for the behavior of one thing in terms of others that are regarded as less complex, or which occupy lower hierarchical levels. We can in this way explain some properties of a molecule in terms of its constituent atoms, and then go on to explain the properties of the atoms in terms of the properties of their elementary particles. But we cannot, in general, do this the other way around. We can account for the properties of mice (to a limited degree) by reference to molecules and atoms, but we cannot explain atoms or molecules in terms of mice.

In the traditional view that machines are simpler than animals, it might make sense to attempt to explain animal behavior, or physiology, in terms of machines. Descartes employed this method, which greatly influenced the thinking of his time, and has had a profound effect upon the subsequent history of thought. Following Descartes, people have successively attempted to explain man in terms of simple machines, clockwork and more complicated mechanical devices and, most recently, in terms of computers. It would seem to be metaphor, however, and not explanation to attempt to account for human behavior in terms of machines built by man for his own purposes. We can explain clockwork in terms of men, but not men in terms of clockwork. The complexity of artifacts comes about because, in a sense, we build into them bits of our own human purposes and knowledge. When we contemplate such artifacts and marvel at their cleverness, we must remember that this cleverness is that of their builders, which has been incorporated into them.

3.4 Artifacts and Their Uses

We have cautioned that our information model is not to be mistaken for an attempt to model language. It is the function of language to convey meaning and, to succeed in this, it must conform to its own set of constraints, its grammar. Natural language is the most general and powerful means we have for the communication of meaning. And, perhaps as a result of this generality, it is not always the most precise or convenient means for dealing with all topics. Arabic numerals are not only a shorthand means for representing quantitative concepts but symbols that conveniently support our ordinary arithmetic operations. An algebraic expression can be easily manipulated using the rules of algebra but may be extremely difficult to process if it is expressed in natural language. The meanings of certain symbols employed in quantum mechanics are not easily translated into natural language nor is there any need for them to be. What counts is whether the initial data and the final results of a calculation can be expressed in the same language in which the observed events are described. Because of the obvious superiority, in appropriate circumstances, of certain symbol systems and calculi over natural language and commonsense reasoning, these are held in high regard. Such symbol systems are sometimes referred to metaphorically as "languages." We frequently hear, for example, that "mathematics is the language of science."

It is difficult to avoid concluding that the use of natural language is a biological phenomenon having a status somewhat similar to such things as respiration, digestion, or consciousness. It is a phenomenon that has arisen through biological *and* social evolution, and has reached its most highly developed form in human societies.[8]

Science too is a part of our artificial world. Among its many disciplines is a composite view of the world as embodied in sets of statements or propositions that have been organized, verified to various degrees, and made public. The truths of scientific descriptions and predictions are supported or confirmed by comparing these descriptions with the corresponding objects and events in the world. When these descriptions and claims are confirmed, or, perhaps more accurately, if we are unable to disconfirm them, they are credited as being provisional truths. As Popper has argued, the strength of scientific claims or theories becomes the greater (a) when these are stated in their most specific and hence most vulnerable forms, and (b) when they have survived attempts at disconfirmation [100]. Our ordinary methods of formulating these descriptions and carrying out their comparisons with nature necessarily involve the use of natural language.

One of the recurring ambitions of philosophers and scientists has been the creation of formal calculi that could be used for carrying out the processing of information as it is used in everyday affairs; particularly in carrying out deductive inferences. The appeal of this stems from the rich successes of mathematics, which can seemingly be applied to raw observations and, through its truth-preserving property, convert them into information in a different and more useful form. For this to succeed, however, as every schoolchild quickly learns, it is first necessary to state an everyday situation in a proper mathematical form. That is, the terms of a situation must first be interpreted. Before we can carry out this encoding, an appropriate abstraction of the situation must be made. Consider the following scenario:

> Johnny Smith took his sister Joan's hand, and helped   (6)
> her to school. He left her at her classroom, and went on
> into his. They differed in age by five years, and one was
> twice as old as the other. This was the first year that
> both Smith children had attended school together.

This is the kind of description we create about an ordinary happening. As such, it is already an abstraction, and it leaves out most of the situation. Provided with this abstraction, it would seem that mathematics might add to our understanding of the story. As we were taught, we can let x = the age of the elder child, and let y = the age of the younger. Taking the facts of the third sentence, we can then write:

$$x - y = 5 \qquad (7)$$
$$x = 2y$$

When we solve these equations, we obtain $x = 10$, and $y = 5$. Reversing the previous encoding procedure, we conclude that the elder child must be ten years of age and the younger one five years. But how old is Johnny? We have no way of knowing. As the reader followed the scenario, it is quite likely that the image came to mind of big brother Johnny taking little sister Joan to school. That would probably be the normal expectation. One might have used this assumption from the beginning and solved the problem by letting x = Johnny's age and y = Joan's age, and concluded that Johnny was ten, and Joan five. Other readers (avoiding algebra altogether) might reason that the younger child, going to school for the first time, was in kindergarten, hence was five years old, so that the children were ten and five, respectively. This solution also fits the data. The assumptions that Johnny is the elder of the two children or that the younger child was in kindergarten might be reasonable ones, but are not supported by the abstraction and can receive no help from mathematics. The possibility of little Johnny leading his blind elder sister Joan to school is nowhere excluded. Mathematics has no equipment *generally* applicable to (6), much less to the original unabstracted situation. It has no tools for dealing with "helping," "school," "sister," or with the idea that it is more likely for older children to help younger ones than the reverse. The techniques of mathematics cannot encompass the totality of everyday situations and, if it is to be used at all, it must be applied to an even simpler abstraction; in this example, to (7). To apply algebra then, we must first perform the further abstraction (and formalization) from (6) to (7) and, in carrying out this step, mathematics itself provides no help. In performing abstractions, we necessarily omit much of the information about a situation and, after we have proceeded from (6) $\rightarrow$ (7), there is no way of reversing our path. We cannot retrace our steps from (7) $\rightarrow$ (6), unless we have made a point of keeping this omitted material in mind. If we were to find (7) written on a blackboard or upon a scrap of paper, there is nothing that would bring (6) to mind. Equation (7) could just as readily arise by considering two planks, one ten feet long and one five feet long, or two piglets, one weighing ten pounds and the other five. This example, trivial as far as situations in the world are concerned, is already too complex to be described by mathematics, and any abstraction of it will leave behind material about which we might hypothesize, conjecture, or argue, using natural language.

Unlike our abstractions of everyday situations in the world, the ones we undertake in physics appear quite different. Here the relevant attributes can be captured in abstractions, and those that cannot be turn out to be unimportant or irrelevant. Thus the velocity with which an object falls toward the earth is unaffected by its color or its cost, or whether someone is standing beneath it. If the law of falling bodies contained such terms, classical physics would still be awaiting the development of a suitable calculus for dealing with them. This circumstance has been stated in the following way by Stanley Jaki:

> Mathematics works in physics because purely physical processes can
> be idealized, and therefore simplified, to an extent that permits their
> handling by mathematical formulas. When it comes to biological

> phenomena, one finds that they are too complex to be represented by ideal cases without destroying their true nature. If, however, their complexity is kept intact, sufficiently powerful mathematical techniques will be lacking for their satisfactory handling. [60]

We will consider some of the reasons for this later.

The impressive successes of mathematics in dealing with the problems of physics has enhanced the lure of creating calculi applicable to problems arising at higher hierarchical levels. The rules of classical (Aristotelian) logic have long been reduced to symbolic form so that, if we are given a series of fact statements, deduction can be carried out by operating upon them in a purely mechanical way. Fundamental insights into mathematics, including a knowledge of its own limitations, have been accomplished in this tradition, the *Principia Mathematica* of Whitehead and Russell being perhaps the best-known example. And just as there are situations in which mathematics provides us with more penetrating insights than does natural language, so there are others in which language is more appropriate than mathematics. Our first task, always, is to select the best tool available. In his book *Personal Knowledge*, Michael Polanyi describes his encounter with the following sentence [97]:

> ...for the variable in the statement form "we cannot prove the statement which is arrived at by substituting the variable in the statement form *Y* the name of the statement form in question" the name of the statement form in question.

He relates that when he showed the passage to Russell, the latter took in its meaning at a glance. Yet this sentence is scarcely one we would expect to encounter in ordinary discourse and, in fact, it was created by J. Findlay [39] as an example of a Goedelian[9] sentence, a subject matter that is capable of being discussed either in comprehensible prose or with the use of symbolic logic. The meaning becomes cryptic when ordinary language is cast in mathematical form rather than in that of conventional language.

3.5 Features of Hierarchical Descriptions

Higher-level objects contain more attributes in their descriptions, either explicitly or embedded, and their descriptions tend to be lengthier and more complex because there is simply more that can be said about them than is the case with lower-level objects. They have more features that are apt to attract our interest or attention. The number of propositions that can be asserted about things in the world is unimaginably large and, in an uninteresting sense, infinite.[10] In speaking of physical objects, however, almost all of the things that could truthfully be said about them would not be worth talking about. If attributes of these objects were to be simply chosen at random they would almost always be irrelevant to our needs or interests.

We first considered the hierarchical organization of matter (as illustrated in figure 3.1) by starting at the bottom and working upward. It has been hypothesized that nature did so as well. At the time of the proposed origin of the universe in the "Big Bang," nothing in this diagram existed. Only after a (very short) period of expanding and cooling did the objects at the lowest level come into existence, and only with further cooling still were molecules formed. The interiors of our sun and the other stars are today still level —8 to —10 affairs. But our knowledge about these things evolved the other way around. People and thought and language necessarily came first, and the organized sense of wonder, which we call science, came very much later. Neither Aristotle nor Galileo had the details we have depicted in figure 3.1 before them, and their consideration of man and the world necessarily started at level 0. This process is still repeated as children perceive, grow up, reason, and begin to talk about things; to them all things are, at first, everyday high-level objects.

We will not explore here the medical importance of these descriptive levels higher than the individual human, and it must suffice to remark that the recognition of their significance to medicine is a fairly recent phenomenon. These higher descriptive levels are now being studied under such names as "medical anthropology" and "medical sociology." It seems certain that we cannot adequately describe or account for such things as diseases without reference to these higher hierarchical levels.

As we begin to ascend the hierarchy, all the simple features characteristic of low-level objects change. The world becomes increasingly complex and rich. As the individuality of objects becomes important, our notion of categories becomes less hard edged and precise. Although we may think of certain kinds of bacteria as being all alike, we know perfectly well that they cannot be—not in the same sense that electrons are. And, when we get to the level of dogs, we find dogs so different from one another that we not only distinguish among breeds but go on and name them individually. Thus, the term *dog* is often too ambiguous to be used without additional details. It makes a difference whether we are being attacked by a Doberman or a toy poodle.

At the higher levels, where we deal with everyday objects, we need a softer procedure not only for naming objects but for forming descriptions as well. Thus, either the description "a big man" or "a very big man" suffices for almost all occasions, and only in rare instances would we care whether the man weighed 240 pounds or 241 pounds. The entire matter of precision takes on a different meaning with high-level objects. It would be pointless to measure a patient's oral temperature to the nearest hundredth of a degree, and we would find a difference of a thousandth of an inch in a person's height to be meaningless. These matters were already understood by Aristotle when he declared, "It is the mark of an educated man to look for precision in each class of things just so far as the nature of the subject admits." What Aristotle's science could not explain (and ours can) was how we go about distinguishing these classes of things.

One concept that emerges from these considerations is that natural language, which has evolved in response to our need for dealing with the objects and processes of everyday life, is "soft" or "fuzzy" in its denotation in order to encompass these things and not miss the intended target. When we state "No dogs allowed!" we mean *both* Dobermans and poodles. Other differences are found as well, when we carefully examine higher-level objects. Unlike the situation at lower levels, where our abstraction or description of a thing and the thing itself seem reasonably congruent, we quickly reach levels where our abstractions and theories embrace matters much less completely. As this happens, we find more and more cases that are exceptions to our rules.

We have remarked that the descriptions in physics lie at the lowest levels. The reader may well ask how it is, then, that we can use physics to account for the properties of macroscopic objects like steam locomotives, which themselves are describable only at higher levels. The answer seems to be that, although we can do this, physics can provide only partial descriptions of steam locomotives. It can deal only with abstractions of the real locomotive, and these abstractions are themselves low-level objects. We can speak of locomotives in terms of energy and momentum and of the strength of materials, using the vocabulary of physics. But this vocabulary does not permit us to speak of railroad-crossing accidents, of the Interstate Commerce Commission and tariffs, of Casey Jones, or of the Great Train Robbery. Our ordinary experience with high-level objects (like steam locomotives) can, however, be abstracted, reduced to simpler representations having a smaller number of attributes, and then described at lower levels where physics does work. This process is nothing more than a reversal of the one by means of which engineers and artisans build locomotives in the first place.

Those having the hope of reducing biology entirely to physics tend to overlook the circumstance that even organic chemistry has not yet been so reduced. Although there is no reason to suppose that organic reactions defy the rules of quantum mechanics, a sufficiently powerful means of employing the latter to predict reaction mechanisms remains to be developed. The abstractions suitable for the representation of organic reactions and for processing with the tools of quantum mechanics do not at present contain everything we need to know. These tools have not yet captured the richness of chemistry. As we ascend this hierarchy, we need different vocabularies, new mathematics (and abstractions), and perhaps even different methods of reasoning as we go.

Finally, the practical, everyday problems with which we deal have properties that depend upon the hierarchical level at which they are formulated. One result of this is the matter of what constitutes a satisfactory answer or solution to a problem. The distinction that I wish to draw here is between "simple" problems (dealing with low-level objects or processes or with the abstractions of higher-level ones) and "complex" problems (which are associated with high-level processes that resist abstraction). The former types of problems typically have a "correct" answer. Answers are either true or false. The questions "What is the product of three and six?" and "For how many people did you set the dining table?" are simple ones involving complete or closed abstractions. Problems arising at high levels do not always have correct answers, and they include questions like "What is the best TV program tonight?" or "How should I treat Disease A in this particular patient?'' It is only with simple or successfully abstracted problems that we can expect to have ''correct'' answers at all. With the others, including most of our everyday problems and almost all medical ones, we can only attempt to find solutions that are ''good enough,'' or ''satisfactory.''

We all believe that we know what the high-level term *man* means, and we would have little difficulty in assigning a one-legged individual, a quadriplegic, or a mentally defective person to this class. But when we cannot agree in particular instances, we must leave science altogether and go to the Supreme Court for a ruling on the nature of the breathing, metabolizing, humanoid object with a flat electroencephalogram (EEG) so that we may legally remove its heart for use in a living patient. How then are we to deal with high-level objects such as these in order that we may properly name them, recognize them, and come to speak meaningfully of them?

4

Information Processes

4.1 Internal Operations Performed Upon Information Statements

We shall now use the information model we have been developing to examine the operations that can be performed upon descriptive statements. We first examine what it is that we mean by the phrase "information processing." We already employed one such information process in chapter 2, where we linked together information statements pertaining to natural objects in order to emphasize the part-whole relationships of objects occupying different hierarchical levels. When we did this, we in no way changed the content (the meaning) of the individual statements. But, by linking them together in particular ways, additional information about the structure of the world was represented. There are many other operations that can be performed with whole information statements, including storage, retrieval, and transmission. Or again, we may wish to compare two statements, term by term, in order to determine their similarities and dissimilarities.

There are also operations that we can perform upon the *contents* of information statements. As we continue the observation of an object, we may extend our description of it by including additional attributes. Or we may take a given statement and eliminate selected attributes in order to enlarge the class membership, that is, we may generalize the statement. The information model suggests that we can perform four basic modifications to the contents of an information statement: we can add or eliminate attributes, and we can add or eliminate nominals. We will see that these four basic operations upon the contents of a statement are associated with a larger number of cognitive activities having such names as generalization, abstraction, particularization, naming, defining, recognition, and classification. The $(N \| A)$ model is useful in exploring the meanings and usages of these terms.

4.2 Naming and Recognizing

The manner in which we learn the names of things and how we forge the mental links between words and objects is sometimes described in terms of a child's learning single "thing" words in the presence of corresponding objects. This process has been recounted by many authors [101, 103] in a form not unlike that provided much earlier by St. Augustine:

> I was now a speaking boy. This I can remember, and since then I have observed how I learned to speak. It was not that my elders provided me with words by some set method of teaching, as they did later on when it came to learning my lessons. No, I learned to speak myself by the use of that mind which you, God, gave me. By making all sorts of cries and noises, all sorts of movements of my limbs, I desired to express my inner feelings, so that people would do what I wanted; but I was incapable of expressing everything I desired to express and I was incapable of making everyone understand. Then I turned things over in my memory. When other people spoke, turned toward this object, I saw and grasped the fact that the sound they uttered was the name given by them to the object which they wished to indicate. That they meant this object and no other was clear from the movements of their bodies, a kind of universal language, expressed by the face, the direction of the eye, gestures of the limbs and tones of the voice, all indicating the state of feeling in the mind as it seeks, enjoys, rejects, or avoids various objects. So, by constantly hearing words placed in their proper order in various sentences, I gradually acquired the knowledge of what they meant. [4]

The words learned through confrontation with objects and the simultaneous hearing or reading of their names have been called "object-words," and the language that comprises them is the "object-language." Such common and necessary words as *when, if,* and *all* are not included in such a language, and it follows that such a language would be incapable of accurately describing our inner feelings. Augustine learned that to do this requires the use of other words, which cannot be learned by confrontation but only through example.

We tend to think of those attributes of a tangible object received directly through the senses as being in some way "primary." These *observables* are of various types, such as color, shape, size, and texture. Each type will take on a particular *value* in a given instance. The attribute of color will take only such permitted values as red, green, or "just like the color of that patch of sky over there." The attribute of shape may take on such values as round, square, or "bottle-shaped." In addition to the attributes that are subject to direct perception, there are others that require the use of instruments such as voltmeters, thermometers, or radiation counters. Scientists consider the pointer readings of such devices to be as valid as direct observation, and regard the attribute-values obtained by the use of such instruments as observables as well.

We have seen that in the case of hierarchical systems the nominal whose attributes are being observed is not itself an observable *at the same descriptive level.* This is not to suggest that nominals are either not subject to observation or that they are invisible. It is simply that when we attend to the attributes of a nominal, with our attention focused upon them, the nominal comes to mind by way of inference or as the recognition of something already known. This is particularly evident in the case of things we can readily talk about but that are not directly seen. We may have a patient complaining of abdominal pain, which has been present off and on for several hours and which is now localized and persistent in the right lower quadrant of the abdomen. Examination reveals that the pain can be aggravated by gentle pressure in this region, and that the patient has a mild fever. The patient's white blood cell count is found to be 12,500 cells per cubic millimeter, and red blood cells are seen upon microscopic examination of the urine sediment. These attributes are those of the nominal "appendicitis," and to have this particular name come to mind is one of the meanings of "diagnosis." Here the nominal is recognized from the set of attributes that is observed. But we do not observe the appendicitis. For it to be regarded as an attribute we must move to a higher descriptive level at which we can speak of the acute diseases of the abdomen. But, when we do that, we are treating appendicitis as an attribute of another, higher-level nominal. Attributes then are the observables we employ when we describe objects or processes. They are Russell's "bundle of qualities." It is only these qualities which we can perceive or observe, and the nominals are the names that stand for particular collections of them.

We can now differentiate more carefully between the apprehension of objects that are directly recognized through perception (the sight of a dog, the smell of cooking bacon, or the hearing of a familiar tune), and the apprehension of objects whose descriptions are being perceived. We have ignored this distinction so far in order to illustrate the results of taking attributes one at a time, as in the creating or decoding (decomposing) of descriptions. When faced with an actual object, our recognition of it almost certainly does not follow the step-by-step, sequential process recounted here. The senses of sight, smell, and touch may present their evidence to consciousness simultaneously. Because they do so, there seems little basis for assuming that, as a general procedure, we can decompose the act of recognition into a collection of primitive and sequential processes.

When, in contrast, we recognize objects not through confrontation but from written or spoken descriptions, recognition would seem to be, at least in part, sequential. If someone is speaking of "the present occupant of the White House," we recognize that the subject is President Reagan and, however this recognition may be triggered, the stimulus for it is a serial sequence of sounds.

We find it convenient to refer to values of attributes as *data*. These are the primary or elementary results of our observing or describing an object or event. This usage conforms to the ordinary meaning of the term in which "data" are regarded as more primitive, as being somehow more fragmentary and less complete than what we mean by "information." More specifically, we would point out that data do not meet the completeness requirement.

These relations can be schematized as follow:

Information Statement

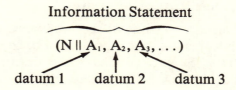

$$(N \| A_1, A_2, A_3, \ldots)$$

datum 1   datum 2   datum 3

The attributes that are apprehended during observation are the data, and our choice of these establishes the descriptive level. We can then always shift our attention to a lower level, which will have the result of nominalizing a given datum or attribute.

Naming or labeling can be regarded as a process that permits us to handle an entire attribute string with convenience and economy. We may call someone's attention to an object either by using its name, or by supplying an appropriate attribute string. We would ordinarily choose the former if we recall the name. If we cannot remember the name ("John Smith"), we are forced to employ the more tedious and less certain method of listing attributes ("The tall red-headed man we met at the lake last summer whose wife, . . . and whose son, . . . ''), and continue in this way until our hearer recognizes the object.

If we present someone with an attribute string, we may be inquiring whether he recognizes the described object (if there is one), and asking him to supply the appropriate name:

$$(? \,\|\, A_1, A_2, A_3, \ldots) \to (N \,\|\, A_1, A_2, A_3, \ldots) \tag{1}$$

This process represents the transactions subsumed under the terms *naming, recognizing,* or *identifying.* Presented in the opposite fashion, we get the formula:

$$(N \,\|\, {-}) \to (N \,\|\, A_1, A_2, A_3, \ldots) \tag{2}$$

In this case, the utterance of the name will, on one hand, call various attributes to mind for someone who is already familiar with the object whose name it is. This act, however, cannot by itself draw attention to any particular attribute. If, on the other hand, our hearer is unfamiliar with the object, we must provide an extended statement so that this becomes a *definition.*

4.3 Distinction, Similarity, and Identity

What do we mean then when we speak of things as being "different"? Our information model permits us to consider this in a more formal way. Suppose we have the descriptions of two objects, N_1 and N_2, each being characterized by a sequence of attributes such that:

$$(N_1 \,\|\, A_1, A_2, A_4, \ldots) \qquad\qquad (3)$$
$$(N_2 \,\|\, A_1, A_2, A_3, \ldots)$$

In examining these attribute strings, we note that N_1 and N_2 are alike in sharing A_1 and A_2. They are unlike, however, in that N_1 has A_4, and N_2 does not, though the latter has A_3, and N_1 does not. Should we then conclude that N_1 and N_2 are different? If we are denied an opportunity for further observation or access to additional data, that is all that we can conclude. If these information statements are open ones, however, it is always possible that further examination of N_1 and N_2 would reveal that they share A_3 and A_4, as well. To deal with this possibility, we must extend our notation to be able to represent the fact that a given attribute was sought, and that it was verified to be absent. We need to be able to represent the absence of attributes as well as their presence. Such absent, or negative, attributes will be prefixed with the tilde ($\sim$). If, in the above example, we had searched for whether N_1 had A_3, and N_2 had A_4, and had confirmed that they were absent, we could then write:

$$(N_1 \,\|\, A_1, A_2, \sim A_3, A_4, \ldots) \qquad\qquad (3a)$$
$$(N_2 \,\|\, A_1, A_2, A_3, \sim A_4, \ldots)$$

We now have a basis, which we did not have before, for stipulating that N_1 and N_2 are, in fact, different. This also provides us with a means for telling them apart even though the statements are open ones and we could go on and say much more about both N_1 and N_2.

This discussion will remind physician readers of the situation that arises upon reading a description of a patient's history or physical examination. A significant clinical attribute may not be mentioned. Should it be concluded that the examiner looked for it and verified that it was absent, or must it be assumed that the describer did not look for it at all? If we are to distinguish between objects on the basis of their descriptions, we need a means for representing the fact that certain attributes are known to be absent. We will see later when we consider the process of diagnosis that the presence and absence of properties play quite distinct roles.

With such high-level objects as living animals, describing them as *living* or as *animals* will entail a host of embedded attributes (referring to such lower-level things as organs, tissues, cells, and particular kinds of molecules), so that the total number of attributes shared by very different kinds of animals will be extremely large. But only a few higher-level attributes (referring to shape or behavior) may be required to tell them apart. Since only one pair of dissimilar attributes (A and $\sim A$) suffices to distinguish between objects, dissimilarity could be viewed as being in some way a stronger condition than similarity. When we have once discovered a pair of discordant attributes, we need not search farther in order to conclude that the two things are different. In a world where we cannot know everything, this method of reasoning permits us to carry out the process of logical elimination, and to conclude with some confidence what a thing is not. This strategy is of great usefulness in medical reasoning. Yet both similarity and dissimilarity occur in degrees, and when we have more of one we have less of the other. Hence:

$$(N_1 \parallel A_1, A_2, A_3, A_4, \sim A_5, \ldots) \tag{4}$$
$$(N_2 \parallel A_1, A_2, A_3, A_4, A_5, \ldots)$$

We might say of N_1 and N_2 in (4) that they are fairly similar from the descriptions given (if we regard the As as being equal in importance). If these descriptions were greatly extended without revealing another pair of discordant attributes, we might then say that they were very similar. However, let us next consider:

$$(N_3 \parallel A_1, \sim A_2, \sim A_3, \sim A_4, \ldots) \tag{5}$$
$$(N_4 \parallel A_1, A_2, A_3, A_4, \ldots)$$

Of N_3 and N_4 in (5), we would probably say that they are quite dissimilar or unlike and, if an extension of their descriptions should reveal that all additional attribute pairs were also unlike, we could agree that N_3 and N_4 were very dissimilar.

In a formal sense, similarity would seem to be reflexive. That is, A would be thought to be similar to B to the same degree that B is similar to A. The evidence (the number of shared attribute pairs) that counts for one is the same evidence that supports the other. Logically we would say that if A s> B, then B s> A, where s> is used to indicate "similar to." Yet it is interesting to find that, in actual situations, a psychological bias may enter into our notion of similarity, and that this introduces an asymmetry. Amos Tversky has discussed this matter in the light of his psychological experiments [130]. The statement "North Korea is similar to China" seems to ring true in a way that "China is similar to North Korea" does not. His explanation for this is that the direction of the asymmetry depends upon the relative richness or completeness of our knowledge of the things being compared. The average Westerner (who has visited neither) probably knows more about China than he does about North Korea. China is more apt to be chosen as the exemplar of the class "Asiatic countries" than is North Korea. It is therefore more likely to be chosen as the standard for comparison. To restate this in terms of our information model, an object with a richer attribute string is more apt to be chosen as the standard for comparison than an object having an abbreviated one. People tend to compare the unfamiliar with the familiar, and comparisons made the other way around sound strange to them. Yet logically there is no basis for this asymmetry.

Another of Tversky's examples can be analyzed in a similar way. To say that "the play was similar to life" makes sense, but to say "life is similar to the play" ordinarily does not. It is generally understood that plays (like novels, portraits, or landscape paintings) are abstractions taken from life, and that they are created by intentionally omitting most of the attributes of actual situations. Thus to say that a portrait is "lifelike" is to praise the painter for having captured some of the more relevant attributes of his subject. But to say that a person or landscape is "like a painting" is to say something that is perhaps meaningful, but is actually metaphorical. It is natural to compare the abstraction with the object from which it was taken rather than the reverse. In ordinary affairs, then, as opposed to logical practice, similarity may be taken as *nonreflexive.*

If two descriptions otherwise the same contain a single discordant attribute pair the nominals cannot be identical. If no such discordant attribute pair is found after a thorough search, we are obliged to regard the two descriptions as indistinguishable *at that stage of the investigation.* In the natural world, the question of the identity of objects does not raise serious problems at the lower hierarchical levels. We can distinguish between so-called identical physical particles, if required to do so, by means of contingent attributes. With higher-level objects, things are quite different. In our ordinary experience we do not expect to find everyday objects to be identical. Among everyday common objects of the same type, we can nearly always distinguish one from another. We may mistakenly take someone else's raincoat or umbrella for our own, but the surprising thing is, given the mass-produced nature of the artifacts of our common use, that this happens so rarely.

Since we can decide whether objects are the same or different by comparing their attribute strings, it might be thought that our model could be used as a tool for deciding such matters. Eugene Rypka has discussed the problem of identifying bacteria in the medical microbiology laboratory from a viewpoint quite similar to the one we have developed [106]. An example of his is the attempted identification of the organism in cases of Campylobacter enteritis. If, by observing the bacterial form, staining characteristics, and growth-temperature behavior, the organism can be assigned to the category Campylobacter, the next step would be to determine the presence or absence of the additional characteristics shown in table 4.1 for the four organisms in this group. The description of each organism (as given by a line of the table) is, in effect, an (N ‖ A) statement.

In an example provided by Rypka, a particular isolate gave the test sequence (S R + + — + + + + +), which corresponds identically to that of *C. fetus* subsp. *jejuni,* and would seem to lead to this identification for this organism. He points out, however, that if this table represents all that is known about these four kinds of bacteria there is no way in which *C. fecalis* can be distinguished from *C. fetus* subsp. *jejuni.* Indeed, there is no basis for speaking of them as "different" organisms.

Rypka provides a second example, one taken from the eighth edition of *Bergey's Manual.*[1] The section on *Hemophilus* describes two organisms, *H. influenzae* and *H. aegyptius,* in terms of characteristics (attribute strings) that do not permit them to be distinguished. On the basis of the cited information, these different names can do no more than refer to the same organism.

Rypka suggests that when bacteriologists acquire data about bacteria they *organize their data horizontally*. That is, they collect data about their objects of study by performing certain observations, and then create the corresponding information statements. Only then, when they have sets of attribute strings in mind, can they compare them with the standard (defining) descriptions of bacterial species and make their identifications.

There are serious doubts whether this account is adequate to describe the cognitive process employed by humans in the recognition of tangible objects. This procedure, however, appears indispensable in the case of invisible objects (atoms) or conceptual ones (diseases). It is also one of the principal ways in which we learn about diseases; that is, as collections of attributes (symptoms, signs, and laboratory findings). Only after this horizontal learning has been completed, and we have sets of such information statements in mind, can we compare them with one another and thus come to recognize, or "diagnose," distinct diseases. In estimating similarity, it is this vertical comparing of attribute strings which is necessary. The utility of this model in explicating the nature of "disease" will be taken up in chapter 5.

Beyond judging the overall similarity of things on the basis of the number of like or unlike attributes, it is necessary to consider whether objects are similar or different in significant respects, or with respect to some theory or rule. Such significant attributes are said to be *relevant*. A donkey may be regarded as being similar to a bicycle in that both are means of human transportation, but this kind of similarity is useful only in the most restricted of contexts. It is not simply the number of shared attributes that determines the similarity of things but the relevance of the attributes in the context at hand. Things are not similar or dissimilar in the abstract, but in concrete situations. What we consider to be relevant stems from our theories of the world and from our experience in dealing with particular situations. We can create descriptions about a pair of identical twins which stress their similarities (physical appearance, stature, or blood types) or which emphasize their dissimilarities (perhaps dress, occupation, politics). Whether we choose one set or the other depends on whether we are trying to help someone tell them apart, or whether one twin is offering to be an organ donor for the other.

Although a continually increasing degree of similarity might seem to approach identity as a sort of limit, the notions themselves are different in kind. Perhaps it is only with abstract objects like Euclidean triangles that it can be said that one object, *A,* is identical to another object, *B.* If we were to grant this, and to further accept that object *B* is identical to object *C,* it would logically follow that *A* is identical to *C.* The property of identity, as with equality (in the sense of Euclidean geometry), would therefore be *transitive.* Similarity does *not* have this property: A may be similar to B, and B similar to C, without requiring that A be similar to C. Suppose we have the three objects A, B, and C, described as follows:

$$(A \parallel a_1, a_3, a_5, a_{10}, a_{12}, \ldots) \tag{6}$$
$$(B \parallel a_1, a_3, a_5, a_6, a_8, a_9, \ldots)$$
$$(C \parallel a_2, a_4, a_6, a_8, a_9, \ldots)$$

Although we can conclude from these descriptions that A is similar to B and B is similar to C, A is highly dissimilar to C. (A s> B, B s> C, but $A \sim$ s> C.) Similarity, unlike identity or equality, is *nontransitive.*

4.4 Necessity, Sufficiency, and Contingency Revisited

In evaluating information statements describing particular objects we may find that their attributes cannot be put on an equal footing. We acknowledge this when we say that some attributes are more "relevant" or "significant" than others within a given context. Necessary attributes are those which a nominal must have in order to qualify for class membership and to be entitled to a certain name and, if we can show that a particular necessary attribute is not to be found in some particular object, we can disqualify it for membership. Its possession of this attribute, however, can only establish its *potential* membership. This is as far as induction can take us. There may be other *sufficient* attributes that have such properties that our finding of even one in an object will guarantee us that the object is a member of a particular class. The possession of necessary attributes confers upon an object the *possibility* of its membership in the class in question; a sufficient attribute confirms this.

Deciding whether an attribute is sufficient requires a much greater amount of knowledge than deciding whether an attribute is necessary. For a polygon to be a square, it is necessary that it have four sides. But a four-sided polygon is only potentially a square; we need to know more about it. For a four-sided polygon to be a square, a sufficient condition would be that its sides were of equal length (to distinguish it from quadrilaterals generally) *and* that the vertex angles were right angles (to distinguish it from a rhombus).

A terser condition of sufficiency would be that a four-sided polygon had diagonals of equal length. To decide whether an attribute of some object is a necessary attribute or not requires that we have knowledge of both the object and its class definition. This information can then lead to our deciding whether membership is possible. To claim sufficiency, however, requires knowledge of all other possible objects in the universe of interest.

A medical example makes this distinction clear. In considering the clinical attributes (symptoms and signs) of different diseases, those of greatest value are called "pathognomonic" (*patho*—disease, *gnomon*—interpreter). The so-called Kayser-Fleischer rings seen in the irises of patients with Wilson's disease are regarded as pathognomonic, and may permit this diagnosis to be made with relative certainty. But if all that were known about this sign was that it always occurred in patients with Wilson's disease, this knowledge would only establish the necessity of this attribute. Encountering this sign would only tell us that a patient *might* have the disease. But the additional knowledge that this sign is seen in no other diseases (which requires that we have a knowledge of *all* diseases) establishes the sufficiency of the attribute and makes it pathognomonic for this disorder. Contingent attributes, in contrast, have nothing to do with either necessity or sufficiency. We have already seen that we can usually distinguish between the necessary and the contingent for low-level objects. It is also at the lower levels that sufficient attributes seem easier to find.

Thomas Sydenham, a founder of modern clinical medicine, already understood much of this by the middle of the seventeenth century. Viewing disease as an internal struggle between noxious influences and the natural healing capabilities of the body, he distinguished among the direct effects of the causative agents on the body (*symptoma essentialis*), effects due to the reaction of the body to these agents (*symptoma accidentalia*), and effects wrought upon the body by the physician in the course of treatment (*symptoma artificalia*). Instead of this last-mentioned term, *symptoma artificalia,* we use the neologisms "side effects" and "iatrogenic disorders," and frequently take them to be twentieth century phenomena.

The processes of naming or generalizing are unconstrained. We are free to name and classify the objects we observe as we wish. We can also choose any name we like, although we must then stick with it.[2] Naming is a device we employ in anticipation of future recognition, and as a convenience in reference. And when we form classes, we are free to do this in any way we wish (as was the case with Jorge Luis Borges's classifications, "quoted" from a "certain Chinese encyclopaedia").[3] We ordinarily attempt, however, to carry this out in a "natural" way in the hope that members of a class so formed will prove to share properties beyond the ones we have selected for the purpose of classification. It is in this hope of discovering laws of nature that we avoid the construction of frivolous classes. The class of objects manufactured last Thursday, or of things larger than a pea, would not be concepts of general usefulness. Instead we attempt to create classes that reflect the regularities we see in nature. The insightful creation of classes is critical to all scientific activity; it has been spoken of as "carving nature at the joints."

When higher-level objects are analyzed, their necessary and contingent attributes become more difficult to distinguish from one another. When first encountered, whales were probably regarded as fish. Their current status as marine mammals became possible only after they had been more carefully observed and described at *lower* hierarchical levels. Only at these levels can we create descriptions of their respiratory, reproductive, and thermoregulatory systems, and thus come to grasp the necessary attributes of these creatures. This shift of attention to lower levels enables us to temper such high-level facts that they "live in the sea" and "look like fish" with the realization that they share many necessary attributes with land mammals and are mammals themselves.

What happens when we turn to artifacts? Matters might appear to become simple again, but we have seen that the apparent simplicity of artifacts is deceiving. Some appear simple because they are models or abstractions of states of affairs in the natural world, in the making of which their creators discarded attributes they believed to be irrelevant or contingent. Indeed, it is the sole aim of abstraction to simplify matters and make them more manageable. The laws and theories of science are examples of this. Some of these constructs, however, have been so highly abstracted that they have had their connections with the world severed. Chess and mathematics may be examples of this. If in some way these particular subjects appear congruent to localized portions of nature, this resemblance may lie in their origins.[4] Other artifacts may appear to be simple because their creators have avoided unnecessary complexity for economic or other practical reasons. But there are artifacts of great complexity that raise some of the same epistemological problems. In the field of technology, for example, we have extremely large and complicated electrical power systems, and very large computers and computer programs. It is well recognized that systems such as these will occasionally display properties that were not anticipated by their designers. Even though humans design and construct such systems, they cannot fully anticipate all their properties. Although these particular systems are vastly less hierarchical, some emergent properties arise as they continue to grow in size. And emergent properties of systems, as we have already seen, are not predictable under theories that are sufficient for the construction of the systems. The emergent properties of artifacts occur as surprises and, as with all surprises, some are unwelcome.

One of the reasons the apparent simplicity of artifacts is misleading has been considered earlier; that is, an explanation of human artifacts requires an explanation of human purposes and activities. Whereas a knowledge of certain laws of physics and chemistry is indispensable to the design and construction of an automobile, these laws alone cannot lead to a complete description of an automobile. Automobiles have all sorts of capabilities and limitations that are not describable with the vocabularies of physics and chemistry alone. The Otto and Diesel cycles are no more central to the operation of automobiles than is the politics of the Middle East. Similarly, to explain a gallows requires much more than a discussion of the tensile strength of rope and a theory of knots. Although the apparent simplicity of artifacts is illusory, some artificial objects are simpler than others by design. With these we may have less difficulty in distinguishing the necessary attributes from the contingent ones. Chess is such an example. We can see that the configuration of the playing board is necessary by definition but that the material out of which it is made is not. The king can be of any shape so long as it is unique, but its moves are prescribed by the rules. Necessity is provided by the rules, contingency by the players.

Some of the classification schemes used with diseases (which are artificial objects, as we shall see later) will be considered in detail in chapter 5 but, because the concepts of necessity, sufficiency, and contingency underlie many of the problems in this field, it is appropriate to anticipate certain of them. The attributes of disease that we call symptoms and signs are among those most characteristically regarded as medical. They are the attributes that cause the patient to consult a physician, and the ones with which the process of diagnosis commences. An important question in the diagnosis of diseases is whether one can distinguish among the necessary, sufficient, and contingent attributes of a disease when they occur at a high level—say, at the level of the entire patient or at the level of a major body region or physiological system. For example, is substernal pain a necessary attribute of myocardial infarction? The answer, of course, is no. The pain in this disorder may occur in the chest, arm, or back or, occasionally, the disease may be painless. The same answer holds for the other symptoms and signs of this disorder. There is no single symptom or sign that is necessarily present in *every* instance of myocardial infarction. Moreover, there is no symptom or sign of myocardial infarction that is not an attribute of one or more other and unrelated disorders. There are, however, attributes of this disease (such as the electrical and biochemical activity of the heart) lying at lower descriptive levels, and some of these are necessary attributes. The electrocardiogram may give evidence of such contingent attributes as an abnormal rate, but it will provide unmistakable electrical evidence for the necessary and sufficient attribute of the disease, the myocardial necrosis due to anoxia (if this involves a tissue volume of sufficient size). At this descriptive level, the necessary and contingent attributes of the disease become separable. Similarly, the measurement of serum enzymes, such as transaminase, may provide independent evidence for the tissue necrosis involved, and confirm the diagnosis.

The fact that some clinical attributes are naturally expressible in numbers has little to do with whether they are necessary or contingent. The importance of measurability may be exaggerated, perhaps because of Lord Kelvin's famous dictum that we really do not understand something unless we can measure it.[5] Attributes that are naturally expressed in numerical form, of course, offer great advantages. For one thing, the measurability of such attributes may help in deciding whether observational data are "normal" or "abnormal." Quantitation may also provide us with a means for assessing the degree of abnormality and, by repeated measurements, for telling us whether matters are getting better or worse. But when attributes are found to be naturally expressible (or *only* expressible) in numerical form, it is frequently because they *are* low-level attributes. And the explanatory power that such attributes provide may be more related to their hierarchical level than to whether they happen to be numerical or not.

4.5 Generalization and Abstraction

We shall now consider performing operations upon the contents of information statements that will render those statements either more *general* or more *abstract*. It is the case that more *A*s are required to describe individuals than are required to describe the species, and more are required to describe the species than the genus. It would be difficult to write an information statement listing all the attributes of a "human," although we have little difficulty in understanding the intended meaning of this word in everyday use. But if one were to succeed in this, the attribute string would be incapable of distinguishing between Napoleon and the reader. In order to achieve particularity with high-level objects, a still larger number of attributes is required, and such statements will have a correspondingly greater information content.

If we wish to reduce the particularity of a statement in order to generalize it, we must eliminate attributes. When we remove an attribute from a description, we reduce its specificity and broaden the class of designated things. At the same time, we reduce the information content. The abbreviated information statement is applicable to more objects in the world, but it asserts less about them. Whenever we remove or eliminate an attribute we perform a *generalization*. We must, however, take great care in deciding which attributes can be omitted if the intended meaning or the truth value of the statement is to be retained. Suppose we have a description of "mammal," and wish to narrow it further so as to designate only "primates." We could do this by adding further attributes relating, say, to improved binocular vision, an opposable thumb, and a more differentiated brain, properties that serve to distinguish primates from other mammals. If we then wished to reverse this process, to take this extended description of primates and generalize it so that all mammals would again be included, it is just those attributes last added that we would have to omit. If we were to eliminate any other attributes, those referring perhaps to properties that may have emerged at lower hierarchical levels, the correspondence between the statement and the object would be lost. We cannot talk about mammals without retaining the idea that we are referring to living organisms. These restrictions result from the hierarchical nature of living things. With nonliving things, the connections between their parts do not run as deeply nor are there as many. A rock split in two yields two smaller rocks. A sheep so divided becomes mutton not two smaller sheep. The process of generalization consists of broadening the description of a class of objects to form a new and more embracing class, and the operation will be valid if the truth value of the description remains unchanged.

The second operation or cognitive process involves the elimination of attributes, and is that of *abstraction*. It differs from generalization primarily in its purpose. Abstraction is undertaken in an attempt to simplify a situation, or in order to describe or model some complex object or process. As we have seen, this is a necessary prerequisite to the use of mathematics in experimental science, and its aim is to convert an otherwise unmanageable subject matter into a manageable one.

The physical concept of a "perfect gas" is an example of one kind of abstraction. The facts that molecules occupy space and may attract one another are ignored (these *A*s being simply eliminated) when we speak of a "perfect gas." The molecules of the gas are then assumed to behave as elastic mass points. This abstraction simplifies the arithmetic, it agrees with certain experiments in an approximate way, and the resulting model systematizes important properties of gases (e.g., Boyle's law), while ignoring properties of (relatively) less importance. In practical engineering, however, this abstraction is useless because it throws away far too much. As Whitehead put the matter, "... an abstraction is nothing else than the omission of part of the truth" [137]. In performing an abstraction, attributes must be discarded with caution lest we throw away something that may be essential to the object in the context of interest.

The reverse process, that of assembling attributes, brings up a different set of risks. The error that one may fall into in the course of assembling attributes carelessly and then assuming that the resulting attribute string corresponds to some object in the world was called by Whitehead the "fallacy of misplaced concreteness." It amounts to the unwarranted conferral of "thinghood" upon an inappropriate attribute string. If we begin by first observing something in the world, and then proceed to describe it, we are developing the information statement from left to right by listing attributes. If we are careful in our observation and description we remain on secure ground. But when we proceed from right to left, we had better be careful that we know where we are heading. If we ask, "What has four legs, a long spiked tail, and exhales vapor that has a mean temperature of 20,000,000°K?" the answer is not "a dragon." There is nothing that can have these *As*—the rules of the world do not permit it.

In describing the notion of an "ecological niche" as a target for the process of biological adaptation, Richard Lewontin has pointed out that it is trivially easy to describe "niches" that are simply unoccupied. "For example, no organism makes a living by laying eggs, crawling along the surface of the ground, eating grass and living for several years. That is, there are no grass eating snakes, even though snakes live in the grass" [68]. One kind of abstraction, the construction of models, is of particular interest to us. Whether models are physical or conceptual, they are intended to be abstractions of real objects or processes. As such, their usefulness depends on how successful their creator is in incorporating relevant attributes and ignoring the others.

A few centuries ago, ship models were commonly built in order to demonstrate to prospective owners a vessel's design features. These models were not intended to sail, some would not even float, and most would be ruined if placed in water. In various museums today they remain a delight to examine because of their craftsmanship. As models they were successful if they demonstrated faithfully the spatial relations of the decks, masts, and rigging of the vessels that were to be built. The ship models built nowadays for testing in a towing tank are quite different. Extreme care is taken in these models to reproduce the precise shapes of the underwater portions of the projected vessels. They are built to float, and are ballasted to do so at the proper waterline, but no particular attention is paid to their appearance. The models may have no decks, superstructures, or masts—their sole purpose is to reproduce, when they are drawn through water, the drag that their full-sized successors will later experience in actual operation. A child's toy boat, which is wound up and placed in the bathtub, is a still cruder model in that it is not an attempt to imitate in an accurate way any specific properties of a real ship. It is successful if it merely floats and moves about under its own power.

These three different kinds of models are each intended to simulate only a few of the very many attributes of an actual vessel. The only way to simulate all of them would be to construct a complete vessel, and that would not be a simulation or a model at all. It is important to remember that models, of whatever kind, are abstractions that have been constructed for specific and limited purposes, and that they leave out substantial portions of the truth. Any properties of the actual object that might be due to these omitted truths cannot thereafter be discovered no matter how intensively the model is studied.

The conceptual models and "thought experiments" of physics have become the paradigm for successful model building. The enormous influence of Newtonian physics and the success of its models have not left biology and medicine unaffected. The reductionist program, the belief that biology can ultimately be reduced to physics, derives much of its support from the successes of physical modeling. Theories based upon the dynamical models of Galileo and Newton were quickly confirmed when they were put to use in such practical affairs as computing artillery trajectories, or predicting the future positions of planets. But, as abstractions, these models fail to account for the behavior of a falling leaf or of a diving bird because of what they leave out.

In medicine and biology we frequently form abstractions for a somewhat different purpose—to typify or exemplify a group of similar, though distinct, objects. Every elementary biology book will display a diagram of a "typical" cell, which will illustrate the cell wall, the nucleus, the mitochondria, and so on. The cell as depicted will be unlike any actual cell, yet it is meant to stand for all of them.[6] Medicine is replete with examples of such models, which we speak of as representing the "typical." Gray's *Anatomy,* for instance, is a compendium of the typical. The first-year medical student quickly realizes that, although the book does not exactly describe the structure of any particular human being, it captures the relevant features of every normal one. For the purpose of teaching medical students, the pathologist will use slides of a "typical" invasive tumor, the radiologist will have a collection of films showing "typical" atelectasis, and students are taught the characteristic sounds of the "typical" murmur of aortic insufficiency.[7] But we do not have in our geometry or chemistry texts pictures of "typical" circles, "typical" squares, or "typical" molecules. There is no such thing in physics as a "typical" magnetic field or a "typical" force. We do not create exemplars or form abstractions with such low-level things because we can deal with them in their entireties. The descriptions of high-level objects, in contrast, would be unmanageable for many purposes unless we first performed an abstraction. When we do this in medicine, the result is frequently the creation of an exemplar; the "typical" case of pneumonia or of congestive heart failure.

Generalization and abstraction are similar in that they both involve the discarding of selected attributes. Yet we distinguish between them for the same reasons that we undertook to make them. Generalization is a process by means of which we hope to make statements about increasingly larger portions of the world without a loss of truth, though at the cost of lost information. As the process of generalization is continued, we succeed in saying less and less about more and more. Whether the information content of extreme generalizations converges to some small but finite value or whether such statements become tautological is a concern that has been raised in criticism of general systems theory in which broad generalizations are espoused [9].

Abstraction is carried out for a different purpose—that of capturing the characteristic features of some state of affairs in a way that will permit us to describe or analyze it. In the process, portions of the truth are knowingly sacrificed, but this is accepted in the hope of discovering a deeper-lying truth. The most important abstractions of science are those that, having stripped away the irrelevancies, provide us with a totally new way of looking at things. These are properly regarded as important discoveries. The great abstractions of Galileo, Newton, and Einstein came about because they had the insight to judge correctly which attributes to retain and which ones to exclude. A major goal of science is to find just these kinds of abstractions. Whatever the means employed may be, the process of scientific abstraction must eventually come to an end. The limit of abstraction is metaphor.

From what has been said so far, no additional emphasis need be laid on the fact that if we err in abstracting a situation we may miss the point of it entirely. When we are presented with the abstraction of a situation, rather than being confronted with the situation itself, our choices are frozen. We may accept the abstractions provided in a clinico-pathological conference case because this is the way the game is played. But we would rarely make a diagnosis with a real patient on the sole basis of a description (abstraction) of the illness provided by a third party. The critical portion of a physician's first encounter with a new patient is in the very earliest phases because it is here that the clinical abstractions are being formulated. We will consider this process in some detail later.

Sir William Osler's insistence that the teaching of clinical medicine must begin at the patient's bedside (a viewpoint that had already been stressed two centuries earlier [82]) emphasizes the importance of this point. An occasional tendency to replace bedside teaching with "chart rounds," to commence with abstractions rather than with actual clinical situations, has drawn much criticism [71]. There are many ways of arriving at the wrong diagnosis, but one of the surest is to begin with an abstraction or model that omits essential facts.

> Models are ways of constructing reality, ways of imposing meaning on the chaos of the phenomenal world. This is not to deny the independent reality of that world but to emphasize that it does not present itself to us organized in the ways we come to view it. The models physicians use have decisive effects on medical behaviour. The models determine what kind of data will be gathered; phenomena become "data" precisely because of their relevance to a particular set of questions (out of the possible sets of questions) which is being asked. Once in place, models act to generate their own verification by excluding phenomena outside the frame of reference the user employs. Models are indispensable but hazardous because they can be mistaken for reality itself rather than as but one way of organizing that reality. [34]

It was pointed out earlier that, as more attributes are included in an information statement, the information content of the statement increases. But there is no more benefit from being in possession of a larger amount of information than we can handle than there is in having more on our plates than we can eat. And we realize, on occasion, that we suffer from too much information rather than too little. The condition referred to as "information overload" is not a fancied but a real hazard. Humans can use information only at a limited rate, and they can only keep a small number of facts in mind at a single moment. The number of different things that we can keep before our minds at one time may be as small as half a dozen. If we are flooded with more information than we can use, the net result is usually an adverse one. In the presence of too much information we may have difficulty in finding what we really need, and we may be diverted by the irrelevant. Abstraction is thus our everyday means for saying enough without saying too much. The current proliferation of clinical data owing to automated technologies and increases in medical knowledge is bringing us ever closer to this disabling state of information overload. The improved management and processing of clinical information is a necessary prerequisite to improving the quality and efficiency of the medical care process.

4.6 Fuzziness and the Limits of Description

In chapter 3, where we considered the hierarchical structure of natural objects, we noted that those at the lower levels had shorter attribute strings than those at the higher levels. There are only a few attributes of a hydrogen atom—still fewer of a proton—which can be observed or measured. Fact statements about such objects tend to be brief. By the time we reach the cell level, matters have become very different. The complexity we find there is so great that the very many attributes of which we may know something provide us with only a partial description.

Although the attributes of simple things are distinct, and more readily distinguished from one another, those of complex objects begin to overlap. Failing to find a single word that precisely denotes an attribute, we commonly discover that we must use several. If we need to distinguish between two fairly similar concepts, we may require extended descriptions of each in order to make the difference clear. A great deal is known about the low-level attributes of the disease phenylketonuria, and this can be clearly described on a single page. Much less is understood about schizophrenia, a disorder characterized by high-level attributes alone, and to discuss these fully requires an entire book.

In a series of papers, Zadeh emphasized the contrast between natural language, and the intuitive means of inference with which we conduct our everyday affairs, and the formal languages (and classical, Aristotelian logic) that are used with such success when dealing with certain abstractions and with computers [141, 142, 143]. He pointed out that natural-language sentences taken at random contain words having "fuzzy" denotations; "John is *tall,*" "It is *quite true* that *many* Swedes are *blond.*" These italicized words are labels of classes in which the transition from membership to nonmembership is gradual rather than abrupt. We find it convenient (if not essential) to be able to use the word *tall* in describing a person; only in special circumstances would we be apt to cite a particular height. Yet there is no specific height that a person must exceed to be "tall," or below which "medium height" is more appropriate. Such fuzzy terms as these are readily understood in everyday usage. In order to appreciate the difference in size between a huge flea and a tiny elephant, however, it is not enough to know the meanings of the words *huge* and *tiny*; we must know something about fleas and elephants as well. As with ambiguity, we can use fuzziness to our advantage because of our commonsense knowledge of the world.

Not only do our everyday descriptions employ these fuzzy or soft terms but, as a consequence, our reasoning, which is based upon descriptions that use them, tends to be approximate rather than exact. Fuzziness appears to enter into our descriptions of everyday objects not through some accidental looseness of language but because of the intrinsic structure of the world itself.[8] Language enables us to articulate sentences (or propositions) in a form that can be communicated and understood, and it enables us to do this economically. But complex objects, which make up the majority of the things we think and talk about in our everyday activities, have attributes that are both more numerous and less sharp or distinct than those of the simple objects, which we talk about only rarely.[9] In describing a person we might say that he or she is "responsible" or "courageous," but these predicates are nowhere near as sharp and distinct as are "mass" and "electric charge." There are situations in which acting responsibly would include being courageous, and others in which the accurate description of an act would require the use of both "responsible" and "courageous." Such terms as these have overlapping regions rather than sharp edges, and it is a matter of ordinary experience that we frequently cannot find single words that correspond precisely to a particular meaning we have in mind.

Zadeh recently wrote, "In a decade or so from now...it may well be hard to understand why linguists, philosophers, logicians, and cognitive scientists have been so reluctant to come to grips with the reality of the pervasive imprecision of natural languages and have persisted so long in trying to fit their theories of syntax, semantics, and knowledge representation into the rigid conceptual mold of two-valued logic." Natural language discourse in its everyday instances indeed displays the fuzzy properties that Zadeh calls to our attention, although it seems to do so much less when simple objects are considered. We can, in fact, discuss and describe atoms and molecules with considerable precision with the use of natural language.[10] And we can and do successfully reason about low-level things using classical two-valued logic. It may be difficult to allocate a newly discovered beetle or bacterium to an existing classification scheme, but there was no difficulty whatever in correctly allocating the newly discovered (transuranic) chemical elements to the periodic table during the 1940s. At the lowest hierarchical levels our descriptive terms do have hard edges, and the transitions between classes are sharply defined. Fuzziness, like ambiguity, is a property that becomes increasingly pronounced as we move to progressively higher hierarchical levels.

It would also appear that, as we deal with more complex objects, we not only require the use of appropriate vocabularies in order to describe them but we may employ different methods of reasoning that are more suitable to these higher levels.[11] Whether or not an atom carries an electric charge is an observable matter, and we can reason from our experimental data using ordinary logic. But whether or not a particular patient displays "weakness" or "anorexia" may not be altogether certain. As a result, we may be unable to decide empirically whether an observation statement containing such high-level terms is true or false, and we may have difficulty in classifying the clinical states that employ them. This issue will have serious implications for us when we consider the process of medical reasoning.

4.7 Information Statements and Inference

In chapter 2 we proposed that an understandable message must contain at least one nominal and one attribute. Let us call such an information statement a *primitive statement*.[12] Primitive statements are created when we observe that a given object (N_1) has some property (A_1) and we write ($N_1 \parallel A_1, \ldots$). Another observer, simultaneously viewing the same object, might note that N_1 has property A_2 and write ($N_1 \parallel A_2, \ldots$). Taking these two primitive statements together, it might seem that N_1 has both the attributes A_1 and A_2, and that the two statements can be combined:

$$(N_1 \parallel A_1, \ldots) \text{ and } (N_1 \parallel A_2, \ldots) \rightarrow (N_1 \parallel A_1, A_2, \ldots) \qquad (7)$$

If ($N_1 \parallel A_1, \ldots$) and ($N_1 \parallel A_2, \ldots$) are both true, will ($N_1 \parallel A_1, A_2, \ldots$) necessarily be true? If the two observation reports were made at different times there might well be problems. We cannot describe the elm tree on the corner in July, describe it again in February, and then combine the two statements.[13] Even if A_1 and A_2 were observed at the same time, is the combination ($N_1 \parallel A_1, A_2, \ldots$) valid? The combining of elementary fact statements may be a risky business when we set about constructing a more comprehensive statement. It will be noted, however, that the resulting statement contains more information, and if the aggregation is a valid one its truth value will remain unimpaired. We must be cautious, however, even in combining simultaneous observations when they are made by different observers. This is especially so when high-level objects are involved.

All observations are made from a particular point of view, not only with respect to an observer's location in space and time but in terms of his use of particular theories, and in light of his reasons for making the observations. The news reports appearing in *Pravda* and in *The New York Times* with respect to some political event might be difficult to combine in this way.[14] These limitations, inherent in all observation reports, should be taken into account when we plan the construction of large clinical data bases in which we hope to aggregate great numbers of independent clinical observations made by different clinical observers, with each perhaps having had different reasons for making the observations. A simple example of this type of problem is the use of archived clinical laboratory data, which are becoming increasingly available in machine-readable form. If only the data values themselves are known, it may not be possible to aggregate them properly without additional information about the individual test methods used, the prevailing ranges of normal values, and the laboratory's quality control performance at a particular time. This ancillary information may be difficult to obtain when such studies are carried out, and it is one of the reasons why retrospective studies are viewed with less confidence than prospective ones. Prospective studies conducted for specific purposes imply a commitment to certain formal procedures in observation, and usually result in more pertinent data than those observations of patients made as a part of routine medical care. The accumulation of computer-readable clinical information in magnetic tape archives can produce a valuable future resource if these considerations are kept in mind during the creation and organization of clinical information. If this collection process proceeds haphazardly (as is frequently the case) its future study will fully tax the skills of the information archaeologist.

The combining of statements is subject to these risks—the inverse process is a much safer one. If we are given the statement $(N_1 \| A_1, A_2, \ldots)$, and we are assured of its truth, we can then perform the decomposition shown in (8) and the process will yield true statements:

$$(N_1 \| A_1, A_2, \ldots) \rightarrow (N_1 \| A_1, \ldots) \text{ and } (N_1 \| A_2, \ldots) \qquad (8)$$

If it is true that "John Smith is a tall man," it is true that "John Smith is a man." The latter statement is said to be *analytically* true. The process of decomposing observation statements leave us on firmer ground than does the process of combining them.

Moreover, the process of decomposition can be applied repeatedly, and in all possible ways:

$$(N_1 \| A_1, A_2, A_3, A_4, \ldots) \rightarrow (N_1 \| A_1, A_2, \ldots) \text{ and } \qquad (9)$$
$$(N_1 \| A_3, A_4, \ldots)$$

then $(N_1 \| A_1, A_2, \ldots) \rightarrow (N_1 \| A_1, \ldots)$ and $(N_1 \| A_2, \ldots)$ and $(N_1 \| A_3, A_4, \ldots) \rightarrow (N_1 \| A_3, \ldots)$ and $(N_1 \| A_4, \ldots)$ or $(N_1 \| A_1, A_2, A_3, A_4, \ldots) \rightarrow (N_1 \| A_1, \ldots)$ and $(N_1 \| A_2, A_3, A_4, \ldots)$, and so forth. This process yields, finally, primitive statements as products.

We can also perform operations that result in the aggregation of Ns. If we are given the primitive statements $(N_1 \| A_1, \ldots)$ and $(N_2 \| A_1, \ldots)$, we can combine them:

$$(N_1 \parallel A_1, \ldots) \text{ and } (N_2 \parallel A_1, \ldots) \rightarrow (N_1, N_2 \parallel A_1, \ldots) \quad (10)$$

With proper precaution, we will suffer no loss of truth here as we do when aggregating attributes. If typhoid is characterized by fever, and measles is as well, we can aggregate this information by creating the category of "febrile diseases," which will contain typhoid and measles. This operation formally creates a *relationship,* and calls our attention to the circumstance that objects N_1 and N_2 both have the common attribute A_1.

There are still other kinds of processes that can be applied to two or more information statements. One important group of processes involves *inference.* The notions involved here are traditionally approached in terms of classical, or Aristotelian, logic. We will briefly examine the simplest of these with the use of the $(N \parallel A)$ model. Suppose we are given that "All men are mortal," and that "Socrates is a man." Let us call this Case I. The first of these sentences can be represented as:

$$(m_1, m_2, m_3, \ldots m_N \parallel \text{mortal}, \ldots) \quad (11)$$

Here we assert that the set of men share the property, *mortal.* Or we may represent the set of all men by M, and write:

$$(M \parallel \text{mortal}, \ldots), \text{ where } M = \{ m_1, m_2, m_3, \ldots m_N \} \quad (12)$$

The second of these premises can be written as:

$$(\text{Socrates} \parallel m_i, \ldots) \quad (13)$$

This statement asserts that Socrates has the property of being a man, and that we would expect to find him in the set $\{ m_1, m_2, m_3, \ldots m_N \}$. This being the case, we can conclude that Socrates is mortal:

$$(\text{Socrates} \parallel \text{mortal}, \ldots) \quad (14)$$

As we saw previously with (9), (12) can always be decomposed. That is, from (12) we may deduce that $(m_1 \parallel \text{mortal}, \ldots)$, $(m_2 \parallel \text{mortal}, \ldots)$, and so on, and we can expect that this sequence will include the instance of Socrates himself. This type of inference, the classical syllogism, is accorded the highest status. If we are assured of the truth of (12) and (13), we can be confident of the truth of the conclusion, (14).

Suppose, instead, that we are told that "Socrates is a man," and "Socrates is mortal" (Case II). We can then combine these as in (7) and write:

$$(\text{Socrates} \parallel \text{man, mortal}, \ldots) \qquad (15)$$

Beyond this step we can proceed no farther without obtaining additional information. But if we observe still other men we may note circumstances that permit us to write the additional statements:

$$(\text{Pythagoras} \parallel \text{man, mortal}, \ldots) \quad (N_1 \parallel \text{man, mortal}, \ldots) \qquad (16)$$
$$(\text{Archimedes} \parallel \text{man, mortal}, \ldots) \quad (N_2 \parallel \text{man, mortal}, \ldots)$$

.

.

.

$$(\text{Napoleon} \parallel \text{man, mortal}, \ldots) \qquad (N_n \parallel \text{man, mortal}, \ldots)$$

Such statements can again be combined so that we have:

$$(N_1, N_2, N_3, \ldots \parallel \text{man, mortal}, \ldots) \qquad (17)$$

We may wonder how many other individual men can be added to these Ns. We could establish that all men born before 1800 are now dead, that is, there are no known men now living who are older than 180 years. We might then make the *inductive* inference that all men are mortal. Such an inference would seem entirely reasonable. It is consistent with our present biological theories. However, as David Hume showed, this inference cannot be logically proven. Although it seems to be an empirical fact, it is not a logical conclusion derived from true premises. So long as there are living men, a counterexample might be found, and it would take only *one*—$(N_i \parallel \text{man}, \sim \text{mortal}, \ldots)$, to invalidate the inference. Induction is therefore a weaker procedure than deduction.

Finally, suppose that we were assured that the remaining pair of statements were true (Case III); that is, that "All men are mortal" and "Socrates is mortal." Is there anything that we might infer from these? Let us say we are given that:

$$(m_1, m_2, m_3, \ldots m_N \parallel \text{mortal}, \ldots) \tag{18}$$

$$(\text{Socrates} \parallel \text{mortal}, \ldots) \tag{19}$$

We may then proceed as before and combine these statements to form:

$$(m_1, m_2, m_3, \ldots m_N, \text{Socrates} \parallel \text{mortal}, \ldots) \tag{20}$$

This statement (20) asserts a relationship between Socrates and men through the common property, mortal. It states that the object, Socrates, possesses the manlike property "mortal," and this at least raises the possibility that Socrates is himself a man. To convince ourselves of this, however, will require additional information. After all, "Socrates" could be the name of my neighbor's dog, and the truth value of (20) would be unchanged. This type of inference has been called by C. S. Peirce, *abduction*. He also referred to it as the making of a hypothesis [94] and, viewed in that manner, abduction is of particular interest to us because of the role played by hypothesis formation in medical diagnosis. Edward Shortliffe [115], in discussing these three types of inference, uses the following example:

If a patient has pneumonia, he will have a fever.   (21)

John has pneumonia.   (22)

John has a fever.   (23)

Using (21) and (22) together to derive (23) is deductive; the combining of (22) and (23) together with other like instances to reach the generalization (21) is inductive. Being given (21) and (23) is a common clinical situation from which we can infer (22)—that John *might* have pneumonia. It is the generation of hypotheses such as this that leads to the formulation of a differential diagnosis. This process will be explored more fully in chapter 6, but it may be noted here that, although hypothesis generation is commonly looked upon as a "creative" act, and hence laden with some mystery, the abductive route to hypothesis formation might seem to be largely mechanical. Let us say we are given that:

$$(\text{Disease}_1 \parallel A_1, \ldots) \tag{24}$$
$$(\text{Disease}_2 \parallel \sim A_1, \ldots)$$
$$(\text{Patient} \parallel A_1, \ldots)$$

We can form the hypothesis that the patient may have Disease$_1$, and we can conclude that he does not have Disease$_2$. But when we say that we are "given" the set of statements (24), these conclusions are already foregone ones and are hence tautologies. The creative feature in hypothesis generation, as it is in the process of forming descriptions, lies with the initial selection of attributes that are regarded as being relevant, and this is by no means algorithmic or mechanical.

4.8 Inference in the Real World

The difficulty with the syllogistic form is that despite its logical strength it does not seem to account for the way in which we reach conclusions, arrive at beliefs, or make decisions in many of our everyday affairs. Most of our everyday choices are not made between alternatives in which one is clearly "right" and the other "wrong" or in which one is "true" and the other "false." The world in which we arrive at beliefs and must make decisions is not divided up in this way. Only after we impose our own sense of structure upon it and generate abstractions of it can we apply such a logic. Many of our day-to-day decisions would not therefore seem to be made by simple deduction. Where, then, does this method work, and where does it not? Classical (two-valued) logic seems to work in everyday affairs in roughly the same kinds of situations in which mathematics works—that is, when a satisfactory abstraction of a situation has been made so that these "hard-edged" methods become applicable. When an everyday situation has been analyzed to this degree, we can say that a "well-structured problem" has been formulated. Only then can the apparatus of classical logic be brought to bear.

With such high-level objects and processes as people and human behavior (which, after all, are the substance of medicine), the abstractions necessary for us to make use of two-valued logic are only occasionally available. In making such decisions as how to treat an arthritic patient, whether or how to punish the guilty, how to educate the young, or whether to continue to treat an irreversibly brain-damaged patient in coma, there are few useful abstractions. These are not, in general, well-structured problems, and, although we may hope to act rationally, we can only rarely claim to do so logically.

Another difficulty with classical logic when we attempt to apply it to high-level, everyday affairs is the difficulty arising from the fuzzy or soft attributes of things. This difficulty does not arise at low hierarchical levels. Here the syllogism works fine. It is a decidable matter, given the description of some object, whether an atom is a hydrogen atom or not. But, as we have seen, stating what is to count as a table or a bird or a person may be much less certain. So in a sense the hoary deduction that Socrates is mortal works largely because we want it to work. That is, it works if we are completely formal about all the terms involved. If our abstractions of the world cannot be formalized, use of the syllogism is in for trouble.[15] This failure is not because the logical apparatus itself does not work, but because we cannot apply it [10].

The premises we have to begin with in medicine will usually contain fuzzy terms, and we may have difficulty in formulating a well-structured problem. We may believe, for example, that we have fairly clear ideas about murder as the intentional taking of a human life. Yet in actual instances, such as a legal defense of mental incompetence in a murder trial, the constitutional question of abortion, or the ethical matter of donor selection in organ transplant cases, the syllogistic form may simply not be applicable because reasonable people may disagree upon the choice of suitable abstractions with which to begin.

At this point it might be helpful to attempt a summarization. In discussing a number of different processes and concepts, it may not have always been clear to the reader where we have been headed. My goal has been to work toward a better understanding of the uses of information in medicine, and if there has been relatively little discussion of medicine so far it is only because there is so much that needs saying about "information" itself.

We have reviewed some of the ideas about how this word can be interpreted, and we have chosen to adopt the view that "information'' is (among other things) something that humans exchange as a means of extending their knowledge. Because descriptions of the world play such an important role in medicine, we have emphasized this type of information and have developed a model for representing the content of descriptive statements. Descriptions of the world bear a peculiar relationship to the world, and when the structure of the world is viewed in a way that reflects its hierarchical properties, the nature of this relationship becomes clearer. When the analyzable structure of the world is so regarded, we find it possible to draw useful distinctions between different kinds of complexity, and among the kinds of descriptions that seem appropriate to each.

We found that in the passage from low- to high-level descriptions, we make use of two undervalued properties: ambiguity and fuzziness. We need ambiguity when we talk about higher-level things because there are simply not enough different words to go around. To be able to speak about the incomparably rich world of everyday experience, we must make words do double duty. At the level corresponding to our daily activity we also need fuzziness, but for a different reason. In order to be able to say something useful about the qualities and properties of ordinary things, we necessarily employ fuzzy attributes because we can rarely find exact ones. And we succeed in our use of ambiguity and fuzziness in ordinary affairs because of the everyday contexts that are shared by speakers and hearers. Sometimes, however, it is these which lie at the bottom of our unresolved controversies.

Granting that the descriptions of low- and high-level objects differ systematically in a number of details, it came as no surprise to find that the manipulation of these descriptions (information processing) also differs for the two cases. Finally, we found that our methods of reasoning, too, must be appropriate to the hierarchical level with which we are dealing. As we turn now to information as it is used in medicine, we will be able to utilize these tools with such central issues as disease and diagnosis.

5

Diseases

5.1 "Disease" and Other Abstractions

The word *disease* is another of those words that, like *information,* we assume we understand until we really begin to think about them. Both *disease* and *information* are everyday words, but they are also high-level terms and therefore suspect. Each may be applied in a variety of situations, and this has resulted in their having acquired a number of different meanings. Although in a commonsense way, everyone—patients and physicians alike—knows what a disease is, few concepts in medicine have caused as much controversy as the notion of disease.

We can begin by considering two contrasting views of disease, each has exerted great influence in the past, and both are widely used today. We shall do this by exploring the nature of the information statements upon which they are based. It is convenient to analyze the notion of disease in this way, because one of these concepts views disease as an entity, as a thing existing by itself, whereas the other fixes attention upon a sick patient and contemplates the clinical attributes that are observed. And, as we have seen in chapter 2, when we cease to think of something as a nominal and begin to attend to its attributes, this redirection of attention triggers a shift in descriptive level. We will then proceed to show how these two views can be accommodated within a single framework, and represented as a network of information statements.

These two contrasting concepts of disease are equally ancient. In the history of Western medicine, both were clearly recognized by the Greeks, although these two concepts did not attain their mature forms until the eighteenth century. In the "thing" or onto-logic view, a disease is regarded as something that is pretty much the same thing whether it is embedded in one patient or in another. Disease is commonly thought of as an isolatable entity having a life of its own. Whether we do so consciously or not, we adopt this point of view whenever we speak of the natural history of a disease, or the course of an illness. This concept of disease has been attributed to Plato, who also provided us with a primitive classification, or nosology. Once "thinghood" has been conferred upon an attribute string it then becomes possible (and irresistible) to go on and classify these things. Thus in the *Timaeus,* Plato divides the diseases of the body into (1) those due to imbalances between the four elements—earth, fire, air, and water, (2) those of the "secondary formation"—marrow, bone, flesh, sinew, and blood, and (3) those caused by breath, phlegm, and bile. His view of disease as an entity is seen when he likens a disease to an ani-mal: "For the course of a disease resembles the life of an animal. Animals are so constituted that there is a set period of life for the species" [95].

Plato's ontologic view of disease results from his fixing atten-tion upon the disease rather than upon the patient. This concept of disease can be formalized in the following manner:

(Disease A ‖ $symptom_1$, $symptom_2$, . . . $sign_1$, $sign_2$, . . . course, . . .)

Under this view, a disease can be described completely in terms of its attributes and without any reference to patients. Indeed, these attributes are regarded as belonging to the disease, and to be able to speak of diseases in this way one does not even need patients. We will refer to this concept as the *nominalist* account of disease.

This procedure is one commonly adopted when we deal with abstract or immaterial things. Even though we cannot point to such intangibles as "inflation" or "summer," we can readily for-mulate the information statements:

(Inflation ‖ decreased purchasing power of money, increase in the free market price of gold, . . .)

(Summer ‖ long days, warm weather, . . .)

These statements may also be true depending on the economic system enjoyed by, or the geographic location of, the describer. In this way we can define abstract objects in terms of their "bundles of qualities," and go on to speak of them meaningfully. These collections of properties, because of their tendency to recur together, attract our attention and invite us to name them. That neither of them is a tangible object causes us little trouble. The ontologic status of these things is similar to that of diseases under the nominalist view.

When such a collection of signs and symptoms has once been given a name, and the disease has become reified, we come to accept it as a thing. We may then go on and speak of its behavior: "...in the short experience [with] *encephalitis lethargica* in this country it is already apparent that its biological properties are altering."[1] The eminent neurologist Hughlings Jackson had earlier made the same point in the case of epilepsy by arguing that:

> The word "epilepsy" should be downgraded, and be used to imply the condition of nerve in sudden and temporary loss of its functions, whether that be loss of sight, loss of consciousness, or "running down of tension," in those parts which govern muscles. [126]

Yet, only a decade later, Jackson was to acknowledge that, whereas medicine as a science required a classification system that advanced knowledge, as an art it needed a clinical classification that was practical, though possibly arbitrary [125].

Hippocrates (or the members the school associated with his name), though accepting that common diseases were entities, and using the popular terms of that time to describe them, is perhaps best known for his case histories. These emphasized, for the first time, the importance of the physician's detailed and systematic description of his observations as he attempted to treat a particular individual's illness. When the sick patient becomes the focus of attention, the resulting view of disease has been referred to by Oswei Temkin as the *physiological* [127], and by H. Cohen [24] as the *biographical* or *historical*. In keeping with the terminology we have developed, we shall refer to this as the *attribute* view of disease, with the understanding that the attributes in this case are those of a particular patient. Under this view, we may observe that John Smith, who is ordinarily energetic, has a normal temperature and exhibits a good appetite displays, in a particular instance of illness, lassitude, fever, and anorexia. These attributes represent the changes he experiences when ill:

(John Smith $_{ill}$ || change$_1$, change$_2$, change$_3$, ...)

John Smith's condition when ill is distinguished by those attributes that represent deviations from his preceding healthy state. And it is those attributes that *constitute* his illness. He will, of course, continue to have a great many other attributes (e.g., being a baker and having brown eyes), which remain unchanged.

In contrasting these two viewpoints it will be noted that causal mechanisms and the desire to understand them are precluded by neither. Plato, the nominalist, also provided us with a physiologic account of disease:

> From sinews and flesh again proceeds a viscous oily fluid which glues the flesh to the bones as well as feeding the growth of the bone around the marrow. . . . When the process takes place in this order the normal result is health, when the role is reversed it is disease. [95]

Yet, unlike the attribute view, the nominalist account does not specifically prompt the question *why*? When a bundle of qualities is recognized and given a name, it seems less pressing to inquire whether there are underlying relations among them. It may not occur to us to inquire *why* summer days are warm, or *why* a lymphoma patient has a fever. Having once named something, we are at risk that we may think we understand it. It appears of less moment, somehow, to inquire into causes under the nominalist view, whereas such questions may become compelling as we reflect upon the abnormal attributes of an individual patient.

The nominalist view would encounter other difficulties as well if, for example, the classification of diseases were to be based strictly upon etiology. As Temkin has pointed out, if we assume that different bacterial species produce different diseases, and the absence of specific essential nutrients or essential genes do likewise, there is danger that specific diseases might be postulated that had no clinical reality.

The attribute view of disease removes this risk of misplaced concreteness: if we observe an abnormality in a patient (setting aside for the moment the question of what we mean by ''abnormal''), there is no more doubt about the existence of the abnormality than there is about the existence of the patient. The attribute view, however, raises a different kind of difficulty, one that was already recognized in Hippocratean times, and later by Galen. These critics did not believe that Hippocrates had provided them with a theory that took into account the individual and that, in the absence of such a generalizing process, each patient's case history would necessarily define a distinct disease. Temkin describes this state of affairs: "Therefore it was concluded, there is no science of the individual, and medicine suffers from a fundamental contradiction: its practice deals with the individual while its theory grasps universals only." The attribute view also leaves us with questions of an operational nature. When is something an abnormality (i.e., what is normal) and when is an individual to be regarded as having a disease?

The Greeks equated health with what was "according to nature," and understood this to arise from a balancing of qualities or humors. Instead of such indistinct things as humors we can now observe structural alterations and measure chemical concentrations and biophysical processes, but the question as to whether these are, in a given instance, normal or abnormal remains. And our ultimate questions about the nature of health lead to our uncertainty about the proper boundaries of medicine.

The tension between the nominalist and attribute views of disease has waxed and waned over the succeeding centuries. The "arch-ontologist" Sydenham (as Temkin has called him), through his painstaking observation and description of diseases, became convinced of the separate and individual characters of diseases to the point where he believed that they could be classified as botanists classify plants. For this insight, Sydenham is honored as one of the founders of medical nosology. But because he lived (1624-1689) before Morgagni's[2] discoveries in pathological anatomy, his ideas regarding the origins of disease were essentially Hippocratean. He seems too, to have had little interest in causal explanations. With the development of gross and, later, microscopic pathology, and the development of improved techniques for physical diagnosis, the possibilities of identifying clinical-pathological connections increased, and causal explanations became more attractive. These developments would eventually set the stage for the reductionist paradigm, which prevails today.

The nominalist-attribute dichotomy of disease continues, and

for good reasons. Neither view alone provides a completely satisfactory way of dealing with the practical problems of medicine.
On the extreme nominalist side we find the public health officer
and the epidemiologist, to whom the name of the disease is the
thing of interest. These individuals work with disease names not
with diseased patients. All occurrences of a particular disease are
looked upon as being the same. Medical economists tend to do
likewise by aggregating instances of illness merely by a name, leading in some instances to the generation of medical cost data that
are completely without meaning. The opposite extreme is exemplified by analytic psychiatrists to whom no two patients are ever
exactly alike, and with whom the search for particularity is a prime
goal. Their clinical descriptions have attribute strings that are
extremely long and, of course, unique. For them, no two instances
of the same disease are exactly alike. The extreme nominalist position thus ignores particularity, and the radical attribute view over-
looks the possibilities of generalization and dismisses universals.

Beyond this controversy over the ontological status of disease,
there are other difficulties in attempting to state what should
count as a disease. We readily concede that a person who feels un-
well (who is ill) and whose complaints can be accounted for under
the theory of a particular disease may be said to have this disease.
But how are we to regard individuals who feel perfectly well but in
whom a physician finds significant abnormalities (the "walking
ill"), or those who feel ill but in whom the physician can find no
"objective" evidence of disease? And, finally, what is to be done
for those who do not feel ill but who are fearful of having some
disease for which neither they nor the physician can produce evidence (the "worried well")?

The outright ill offer few problems, and we will consider the
conventional ways in which their afflictions can be analyzed and
described. The individual without symptoms in whom an abnormality is found (a questionable mass in the breast, a worrisome-
appearing skin lesion, an enlarged lymph node) might not be said
to have a disease because of these findings alone. Ordinary common sense as well as medical prudence require an explanation for
such findings in order to exclude disease.

A different category of illness includes the obviously distressed
patients for whom medical investigation reveals no evidence of
what is commonly referred to as "organic" disease. Treating such

patients as these has long been a difficult problem for physicians. These patients represent an assortment of situations ranging from the patient with vague symptoms and emotional complaints in whom a frontal lobe tumor will eventually be found to the unhappy patients displaying no "organic" disease now (nor will they in the future) and who will eventually be labeled as having personality or maladjustment problems. The "worried well" form an appreciable group of patients to be found in physicians' offices and in clinics, and Sidney Garfield has properly emphasized the need for their recognition and management [144].

Still different questions are raised by patients having complaints explainable by clear and objective evidence, but for which the word "disease" does not seem quite fitting. Does the individual who has had a hemostat inadvertently left in his abdomen during surgery have a disease? If disease is to be regarded as a change in physiological state, is a person who has recovered from chicken pox and is now immune to it, diseased? He is demonstrably different now. Or is disease to be simply equated with the loss or reduction of some physiological function? If so, are the voluntarily sterilized diseased? In order to deal with such questions, the term *medical condition* is commonly used to refer to circumstances in which the term *disease* does not seem appropriate. The current edition of the *International Classification of Diseases* (ICD)[3] provides a uniform classification scheme for diseases, injuries, impairments, symptoms, and causes of death, and in its foreword the editor looks forward to a future revision as "an International Classification of Disease, Disorders, and Health Problems." This continuing extension of what counts as disease, or what needs classifying, results in part from the growing demand for medical information by government bureaus, the health insurance industry, medical specialty organizations, hospital associations, environmental health and safety authorities, epidemiologists, and health system administrators. Also contributing to this demand is the increasing use of computer-based information systems, which now make it feasible to process these detailed and voluminous health data once they are recorded. Although in earlier times it may have sufficed for officialdom to note whether a man died from "natural causes" or from "violence," we can now in the official record distinguish between an accident victim who sustained his injuries while riding an animal during the latter's collision with another animal, and a rider whose mount collided with a pedal cyclist (ICD-9-CM).

Finally, there is the common but vague view of disease as a state that is, somehow or other, just "different" from that of health. Since this view is, in practice, defined in terms of what is regarded as usual or "normal" for a member of a particular population, it results in a concept of disease arising from a statistical procedure. Such an approach has obvious limitations.[4] Nevertheless, as increasing use is made of quantitative clinical and laboratory methods, the only practical means available to us for analyzing the observed data are statistical ones.

Because our interest here lies with the patient and the physician, we will proceed by viewing disease as something happening to and experienced by the patient, which is investigated, described, and treated by the physician. In so doing we will continue to contrast the nominalist view of disease, which appears to underlie such common notions as "diagnosis as recognition" or "diagnosis by pattern matching," with the attribute view of disease, which implicitly embodies a search for causes and a desire to explain. We will see that whereas the former tends to regard disease as occupying a single descriptive level, the latter involves the creation of information statements describing affairs at a number of different hierarchical levels. We will also see that, although neither view alone provides the physician with a method applicable to all instances of disease, the two views can be combined into a single representation which is complete.

The possibilities of accomplishing this will become apparent by examining a well-known, if nonmedical, example. In the introduction to his Gifford Lectures, Eddington wrote of his "two tables" [33].[5] The first of these was the ordinary, visible, and substantial one that supported his writing paper and inkwell. The other he termed his "scientific" table, and he went on to point out that it consisted only of numerous electric charges rushing about at high speeds, and that it was nearly all empty space. Eddington then asked, "Which is the real table?" and he proceeded to answer, "The second." His question has subsequently been discussed by many writers. Ernest Nagel, for example, discusses it and disagrees with Eddington by pointing out that the word *table* signifies an experimental idea that does not occur in the language of electron theory [90]. This portion of Nagel's argument I take to be sufficient to support the refutation that there is only one "table," namely Eddington's first one. Because the example of Eddington's table illustrates so clearly the nature of the descriptions of hierarchical systems, it is worth examining in some detail, keeping in mind that what we discover will be equally applicable to the case of disease. With the latter, we will be asking, Which is the real disease, the nominalist's "bundle of qualities" or the string of patient attributes?

Now a table (Eddington's or anyone's) is an object which we ordinarily describe in terms of size, shape, the material out of which it is constructed, the use to which it is put, and its finish and appearance. The word "table" is part of the vocabulary we use in speaking of articles of furniture. Suppose that we have a wooden table and we consider it at the next lower level of description, that of its major components. It might have a top planked with quartersawed oak, and turned oak legs fastened to the top in a particular manner. Examining the table more closely, we could describe the grain of the wood and perhaps infer something about the growth, age, or size of the tree(s) from which it was made. At a lower level, perhaps microscopically, we could go on to describe the cellular structure of the wood, and by suitable tests we could determine other physical properties of the lumber. As we did this, we would soon find ourselves at levels where "furniture words" were no longer applicable. At such levels there are no tables, just wood. We can move on down to a still lower level and find out something about, say, its cellulose and lignin content and learn about its other chemical properties. Here we can no longer use the languages of either "furniture" or of "lumber." We may then proceed and inquire still more deeply and, only after three or four more levels, would we finally reach Eddington's table consisting of electrons and atomic nuclei.

Although it is a disconcerting leap to proceed directly, as Eddington did, from his first table to his second, it becomes very much less so if we systematically descend these hierarchical levels one at a time. The conceptual contacts between any two adjacent levels in our description of tables are numerous, and we can find more or less satisfying explanations for the behavior of things at one level in terms of the one immediately below it. It is a much more difficult matter, however, to account for the properties exhibited at one particular level from the behavior of its constituents described at three or four levels below, unless we examine the intervening ones. And as we proceed from the top to the bottom of this network of descriptions, certain processes predictably set in. The high-level terms (like *table, leg, top*) are both ambiguous and fuzzy, but they become less so as we proceed downward. The word *table* itself (meaning an item of furniture) raises well-known and difficult questions of definition, and it is by no means clear how we actually go about deciding whether some object is a table or not. We might ask whether an obvious feature like having legs is a necessary or contingent property. There are objects that we would regard as tables that have no legs (being supported by brackets, or suspended), one leg, two legs, three legs, and so on, up to a score or more of legs. Counting legs turns out to be of little help. What of its function as a support for other objects? If we consider that, how do we then tell a table from a desk, a bench (e.g., a workbench), a stand, a shelf, or a tripod? These questions arise expectedly because of the ambiguity of the terms we use with such high-level and everyday objects. At lower levels, our terms become sharper; *wood* has a fairly well-circumscribed meaning, though we might have trouble with a few objects, such as a rattan table, or tables made of compacted sawdust and wood chips. At the level of cellulose, matters become sharper still. And, finally, at the level of atoms or elementary particles, our descriptions become sharp and precise. Only here do word and object point uniquely to each other. And, with the decreased ambiguity and fuzziness at lower levels, we find it easier to distinguish between the necessary and contingent properties of the terms. Eddington's tables, and his question, "Which is the real one?" will have their counterparts as we now turn to disease.

5.2 Disease as Name

The concept of disease as a "thing" is so widespread in medicine and it serves so many practical ends that it deserves a full hearing. Since there is no completely satisfactory definition of what constitutes a disease, diseases cannot be exhaustively listed or counted. We can, however, estimate the approximate number of diseases or medical conditions that medical nosologists regard as distinct entities, and which public health agencies employ in recording their statistics. If one examines ICD-9-CM, it will be found that the number of codable conditions is something on the order of 25,000. In addition to common diseases and their variants, there are such detailed conditions as the fractures of particular bones (and of particular parts of particular bones) and the loss of function of certain motor nerves. Thus a cross-eyed patient may be simply said to have "strabismus" (in ICD, coded as 378), or this may be further described as "paralytic strabismus" (378.5). But one can proceed still farther and describe it as "third or oculomotor nerve palsy, total" (378.52). The first statement stands as an example of disease (or condition) as a name; the common expression "cross-eyed" being translated directly into medical terminology as "strabismus." But this is a crude description stating only that there is a disorder of binocular eye movements and adds nothing about the nature of the abnormality; that is, it does not distinguish among the several types of strabismus that may be readily recognized. Finally, the continued study of a patient with strabismus may reveal a specific physiological deficit; in the example used here, the loss of function of a particular motor nerve. At this point, our view of the entire matter has begun to shift. We no longer think so much that Tommy Jones has the disorder or condition strabismus, but that he has a third-cranial nerve palsy. And once we begin to think along such causal lines we may wonder about the cause of the nerve palsy; does it result from some self-limiting and perhaps reversible process, or is it a permanent loss of function? Here we began with a named disorder (strabismus) that is readily thought of as a thing. In the ophthalmology departments of our medical centers there may be "strabismus clinics," and ophthalmologists will hold "strabismus rounds." Yet the patients who find themselves in these clinics or are the subjects of these discussions will have a number of different neurological, anatomical, or neuromuscular defects, which have arisen through a variety of developmental or perhaps environmental factors. It is the nature and the origins of these defects which we seek. Since it is in the early stages of causal chains that medical treatment is most effective, physicians prefer to treat causes rather than effects. While we began by thinking of strabismus as a thing, we ended by focusing upon particular functional deficits and their causes.

Let us now turn to a totally different sort of disease, the group of disorders known as the schizophrenias. Under one classification [2], these have been divided into ten subtypes, each being provided with its own name. The listed attributes of these diseases, which provide the sole basis for their diagnosis and classification, are all signs of disturbed or abnormal behavior. There are at present no known physical signs or visible lesions of these diseases, no standard laboratory tests are helpful, and no tissue or cellular abnormalities are to be found by the pathologist at autopsy. A few of the attributes used in describing these disorders are "emotional response shallow," "restlessness," "posturing," "unpredictable behavior," "staring," "gesturing," "confusion," "scornful," "sarcastic," and so on. When we reflect upon the fuzziness and contingency of these attributes, we are not surprised that some physicians have been deeply troubled by the ontologic status of these diseases. Thomas Szasz in particular has taken a radically destructive view of the concept of mental illness, and has pronounced that "...disease or illness can affect only the body" [123]; hence there can be no mental illness.[6] He concludes that "...'mental illness' is a metaphor." Despite Szasz's surprising Cartesian argument, mental diseases raise not only ontological questions but present us with social imperatives as well. For the individual who insists that he is a poached egg, society will inevitably create a category and a name, and for one who attempts to jump from a tall building, it will insist on intervention and restraint.

No single attribute enumerated above for the schizophrenias would, when taken alone, suffice for the diagnosis of this disease. Most normal people will display one or more from time to time, and few schizophrenic patients will display all of them. All of these attributes are contingent with respect to this diagnosis. The diagnosis of schizophrenia must be made on the basis of accumulated observations and careful judgment. Its correctness in borderline cases will always be subject to doubt. Nevertheless, moderately severe cases will be diagnosed by most physicians, and seriously affected patients will be recognized by laymen.

Now the important difference between strabismus and schizophrenia is that the former can be described at several different hierarchical levels, and it is known to involve such tangible things as particular nerves, specific muscles, and the motions of the eyes. There is also a certain causal plausibility by means of which these attributes, lying at different levels, can be connected. In contrast, the description of schizophrenia lies at a single, very high level where fuzziness and ambiguity of reference are the greatest, where explanations are at present unsatisfactory, where the sufficiency of attributes of the disease is not established, and certainty in diagnosis is elusive.

It was not long ago that many of the common medical diseases had an ontologic status not much more secure than that of the schizophrenias. To be sure, they had more tangible (physical) attributes; the combination of fever, cough, production of blood-streaked sputum, pleuritic pain, and rales has long meant pneumonia. And at one time the disease pneumonia called for treatment with mustard plasters or other measures of doubtful value. The understanding of pneumonia and its treatment began to improve with the development and acceptance of the germ theory of disease. When pneumococcal antisera and, later, antibiotics became available, the diagnostic goal became that of identifying the causal agent so that specific therapy could be initiated. The high-level attributes, the symptoms and signs of this disease remain the same today, but the therapeutic aim is no longer to treat the pneumonia. Instead, we treat (if possible) the infectious agent that has been identified and is believed to cause the pneumonia. When we speak of *specific* therapy, we are most likely found to be referring to lower-level things, to matters lying at the organ, cell, or molecular level. Here, the disease process can be confronted in its early causality. Nonspecific or *symptomatic* therapy is concerned with the alleviation of abnormalities lying at higher levels, and it is these, of course, from which the patient suffers. Just as we can distinguish high- from low-level abnormalities so can we contrast high-level with low-level treatment.

In chapter 4, we recounted one learning process that is closely related to the process of naming. We are able to learn that a particular object is a "ball" or a "mitral valve" by apprehending an appropriate set of attributes, and we can then distinguish those objects from "blocks" and "tricuspid valves" by comparing their respective attributes. One of the principal methods by means of which we learn about diseases involves just this process. We first learn about diseases that are poorly understood in pathogenetic terms, and about syndromes generally, with a collection of attributes. Reiter's Syndrome is understood to be the name applied to the attribute string "urethritis," "arthritis," and "conjunctivitis." When we find a patient to have one of these attributes we may look for the others. But even with disorders where a more complete pathophysiological account is available, as with aortic insufficiency, it is frequently the attributes "high-pitched diastolic murmur along left sternal border," "Austen-Flint murmur," "Corrigan pulse," that lead to a clinical diagnosis. We first learn many things in clinical medicine in this horizontal or single-level fashion. And then when we wish to apply this knowledge to distinguish among similar diseases, we find the next step more difficult. This is the problem faced by the third-year medical student who has learned about diseases in terms of their attribute strings. Having learned about diseases individually, he or she must then begin the more difficult vertical process of sorting through the respective attribute strings in order to compare, contrast, and distinguish one disease from another. But it should be noted that if our knowledge of diseases were organized exclusively in pathogenetic (causal) terms it would be awkward to talk about them, and difficult to recognize them at the bedside.

5.3 Clinical Attributes As Disease

Although certain attributes of a sick patient were taken in ancient times for the disease itself (a flushed, warm, perspiring patient was said to "have the fever"), it was the discoveries of nineteenth-century pathologists that first made the attribute view an appealing one. In 1849, Rudolf Virchow, the founder of cellular pathology, argued:

> ... the destruction of the ontological conception of disease is also a destruction of ontological therapy, of the school of *specifics*. The subjects of therapy are not diseases but conditions; we are everywhere only concerned with changes in the conditions of life. Disease is nothing but life under altered conditions. (in *Die Einheitsbestrebungen in der wissenschaftlichen Medizin*)

And these altered conditions occurring in disease frequently manifest themselves, as Virchow would later describe in his *Die Cellularpathologie* (1858), as the altered attributes of tissues and cells. The power and attraction of the attribute view lay in the certainty afforded by those tangible abnormalities upon which multiple observers could agree. Such directly apprehended attributes as trauma (fractures, dislocations, burns) and congenital malformations (harelip, polydactly) have long been looked upon *as consti-tuting* the disease and continue in that role today. In these instances, the confirmation of a patient's abnormal attribute(s) entails the diagnosis of the disease. A necessary (and sufficient) attribute of the condition "fracture" is the recognition that the continuity of some structure, commonly a bone, has been disrupted. This may be obvious from a brief glance, it may require a careful physical examination, or it may be detectable only upon an X-ray examination. But without evidence of the attribute "fracture" there can be no diagnosis of the condition "fracture."

The diagnostic leverage afforded by the attribute view has increased greatly during the present century because modern technology has provided us with the means (physical, chemical, and biological testing) for observing attributes of the sick patient at continually lower hierarchical levels. These methods of observation provide a means for distinguishing between those attributes that are necessary to the diagnosis of a disease and others that are merely contingent. The diagnostic confidence afforded by pathognomonic findings (being regarded as specific for a particular disease) has been recognized since the early nineteenth century. Such attributes are sufficient for a diagnosis. Once only rarely available (and traditionally referring to symptoms or signs), such pathognomonic or specific findings are being increasingly employed in diagnosis as physiological and biochemical research reveals them. They are particularly useful when they provide lower-level explanations of the etiology or pathogenesis of diseases. It will be understood, however, that necessity and specificity are different kinds of things. Some specific findings may be so for purely definitional reasons; "hypertension" is the disease displayed by a patient whose blood pressure measurements are repeatedly elevated. The finding of increased blood pressure (measured under specified conditions) thus entails the diagnosis "hypertension." Similarly, "heart block," "agammaglobulinemia," "cystinosis," "hypovitaminosis A," and many others are diseases that take their names from a single abnormal attribute, which can be directly measured and the confirmation of which is sufficient for the diagnosis. While such findings are specific and sufficient (pathognomonic), they are so in a tautologic sense. These disorders all show other associated clinical findings as well, most of which are contingent. What we refer to as specific disease attributes are therefore necessary ones, although necessary attributes need not be specific.

The regarding of attributes as diseases has had a powerful attraction (this is the way in which we view machines) because of the explanatory power that it may provide. A practical limitation to this approach is that only certain diseases are presently understood in enough detail to make the procedure a useful one. A more important consideration is the fact that patients seek medical help not because they have lower-level abnormalities (enzyme or nutritional deficiencies, biochemical abnormalities, or organ or tissue pathologies) but because they have aches or pains or other disturbances of higher-level functions from which they directly suffer. A patient cannot directly experience abnormalities of blood glucose concentration, although he or she may experience faintness or hunger or be abnormally thirsty. It is their symptoms that patients want physicians to set right. And all that we can mean by "treating the patient as a whole" is no more than insisting that attention be paid to abnormalities at whatever level they are to be found. Since both the nominalist and attribute views of disease suffer from the limitations we have discussed, we will next see whether features of both can be combined in a way that will overcome these shortcomings.

5.4 A Hierarchical Model of Disease and Illness

We have seen that the descriptions of natural hierarchical systems display systematic properties and, if we have sufficient information about them, they can be interconnected to form what we will call attribute lattices, or knowledge networks. We have also seen that these descriptions must be carried out with the use of languages appropriate to the hierarchical level involved. We will now employ these same procedures with diseases.

The patient abnormalities that we examine one at a time, so to speak, in the attribute view of disease, or that we examine as a bundle of qualities apprehended collectively in the nominalist view, occur, not just generally, but at particular hierarchical levels. Some symptoms like anxiety, fever, or anorexia are not experienced in a particular part of the body or in a single organ, but "all over." In contrast, the pain of angina pectoris is experienced in certain body parts and not in others, even though it is not experienced in the heart itself where its origin lies.

Let us adopt the following scheme of hierarchical levels, as a means of illustrating this process:

TABLE 5.1

Hierarchical Levels of Medical Descriptions	
Level 0	Patient as a whole
Level —1	Major patient part: e.g., chest, abdomen, head
Level —2	Physiologic system: e.g., cardiovascular system, respiratory system
Level —3	System part, or organ: e.g., heart, major vessels, lungs
Level —4	Organ part, or tissue: e.g., myocardium, bone marrow
Level —5	Cell: e.g., epithelial cell, fibroblast, lymphocyte
Level —6	Cell part: e.g., cell membrane, organelles, nucleus
Level —7	Macromolecule: e.g., enzyme, structural protein, nucleic acid
Level —8	Micromolecule: e.g., glucose, ascorbic acid
Level —9	Atoms or ions: e.g., sodium iron

If we examine the vocabulary used in *Current Medical Information and Terminology* (CMIT) [2] for describing symptoms, we find that it is possible, in an approximate way, to assign those terms to the levels in table 5.1. For example, the word *pain* is most frequently used by a patient to describe a particular kind of unpleasant sensation experienced in a body part, or perhaps to the body as a whole: "I hurt (ache) all over." Or, it may be ordinarily ascribed by the patient to a physiological system, or even to an organ (pain in one eye). We will therefore assign this term to the range of levels 0 through —2, since "pain" is a word in the language used by the patient to describe matters at these levels. Reasoning in a similar manner, we will allocate "nausea" and "vomiting" to level —2 or —3, since the patient experiences these phenomena as being associated with the upper portion of the digestive system. If we continue on with the more frequent terms employed as symptoms, and assign them to these hierarchical levels, we obtain the results shown in table 5.1.

We shall now consider some specific diseases, employing the disease attributes used in CMIT. (These attributes in CMIT were, in turn, taken from the descriptions of diseases provided in standard medical textbooks.) In order to define the disease *Manic Depressive Illness (Manic phase)*, CMIT employs thirty-four different attributes, all being symptoms or signs, and all are behavioral attributes. All are level 0 terms. No other characteristics of the disease are provided, or indeed known. We may then arrange these terms to form the attribute lattice (or knowledge network) corresponding to the definition of this disorder, which is shown in part in figure 5.1. Since no lower-level attributes are known, the lower levels are unoccupied, and the description occurs at a single high level.

Level 0   assertiveness, excitement, insomnia, irritability, . . .
Level —1   _____
Level —2   _____
Level —3   _____
Level —4   _____
Level —5   _____
Level —6   _____
Level —7   _____
Level —8   _____
Level —9   _____

Figure 5.1. Attribute network for manic depressive illness.

Since each listed attribute of this disease is a behavioral one, the terms themselves are words belonging to the vocabulary with which we describe patients as a whole (level 0). Neither a part of a patient nor an organ or tissue can be *assertive* or *wakeful*. It will also be noted that these disease attributes are fuzzy ones. (What is the precise boundary separating insomnia from a "normal" degree of sleeplessness or restlessness? What is the exact demarcation between excitement and enthusiasm?)[7] It is also the case that each of these attributes is contingent, and that a diagnosis can be made in the absence of one or more of them. Psychiatric disorders, in large part, have representations similar to this one, given our present understanding of mental illness. This representation is, of course, not intended to suggest that these attributes are all that need be learned about depression, or to claim that these symptoms are in some way free-floating at this high a level and without any causal means of support. It simply represents the clinical description of the disorder as it is currently known, and underlines what needs to be learned.

As an example of a quite different kind of disease, one having attributes lying at several distinct descriptive levels, we will consider the uncommon tumor, pheochromocytoma. Again, using the disease attributes taken from CMIT, we can form the representation shown in figure 5.2.

Level 0	nervousness, tremulousness
Level —1	headache, dizziness
Level —2	hypertension, polydipsia, polyuria, blurred vision
Level —3	nausea, vomiting, dyspnea
Level —4	dilated pupils
Level —5	cells large, irregular, or polyhedral; granular cytoplasm
Level —6	_____
Level —7	_____
Level —8	increased epinephrine, norepinephrine, VMA, metanephrine
Level —9	_____

Figure 5.2. Attribute network for pheochromocytoma.

It will again be seen that it is the higher-level (levels 0 through —3) contingent attributes that are experienced by the patient, and which make the patient "ill." All of these higher-level attributes are those of other diseases as well, and none of them taken alone would permit us to make the diagnosis of pheochromocytoma. It will be seen too that we can account for the occurrence of some findings in terms of others on the basis of known physiological mechanisms. The relationships among these attributes reflect underlying biological laws, and we can trace causal paths among them based upon our knowledge of these laws.

Again, the higher-level attributes of this disease are fuzzy and ambiguous but, as we move downward, "blurred vision" seems less so than "nervousness," and "dilated pupils" is a still more objective and certain finding upon which multiple observers might agree. The level —8 attributes, in contrast, are definite and sharp and can be positively identified and measured by suitable tests. The diagnosis of this disease is most frequently made by first suspecting it on the basis of higher-level attributes (usually as a cause of unexplained hypertension), and then by performing those chemical tests upon a urine specimen which will reveal the distinctive and diagnostic level —7 abnormalities. These are among the necessary attributes and would ordinarily be sufficient for the diagnosis, although histopathological confirmation would be sought following the surgical treatment of the disease.

As a third example, we will consider the common disease, chicken pox (varicella). We can assign the attributes of this disease to their appropriate levels and obtain:

Level 0	anorexia, malaise
Level —1	headache; lesions on trunk, spreading to face, scalp
Level —2	lymphadenopathy
Level —3	pruritus; red papules becoming clear, umbilicated
Level —4	_____
Level —5	leukocytosis, epithelial cells with intra-nuclear inclusions
Level —6	varicella virus
Level —7	_____
Level —8	_____
Level —9	_____

Figure 5.3. Aspect lattice for chicken pox (varicella).

Here again the attributes are distributed over a number of hierarchical levels, and include features that can be experienced only by the patient, others that can be observed by the physician, and some that require laboratory procedures for detection. Since relatively little is understood about the detailed causal mechanisms in viral diseases, the connections between the attributes in varicella are less complete than they are in pheochromocytoma. Our knowledge of the biological laws accounting for the pathogenesis of viral disorders does not yet permit us to indicate all the causal connections, although the abnormalities themselves are easily recognized, and may be assigned to appropriate levels.

The representations shown in figures 5.1, 5.2, and 5.3 illustrate several of the advantages of representing our knowledge of diseases in the form of such descriptive networks. First, by systematically assigning attributes to the hierarchical level at which their referents emerge, the nature and extent of our knowledge of a particular disease is made explicit. Next, this helps to identify the points at which therapeutic intervention may be employed, and clarifies the distinction between symptomatic and specific treatment (urging us to treat both the patient and the disease). This representation further invites us to distinguish "downward causality" ("stress induces the increased production of gastric acid") from "upward causality" ("increased gastric acidity favors ulcer formation"). It also suggests that the process of pathogenesis usually involves two or more different levels. A cause that can be allocated to one level frequently appears to have effects lying at different levels.

The knowledge network model of disease also permits us to characterize the several categories of patients remarked upon earlier: (a) the patient with no "organic" disease, (b) the patient with asymptomatic disease, and (c) the "sick" patient. These are represented in schematic form in figure 5.4.

(a)   (b)   (c)

Level 0 A_1, A_2, A_3, A_4	0	0 A_{10}
Level —1	—1	—1
Level —2	—2	—2 A_{11}, A_{12}
Level —3	—3	—3 A_{13}
Level —4	—4	—4
Level —5	—5	—5
Level —6	—6	—6 A_{14}
Level —7	—7	—7
Level —8	—8 A_5, A_6	—8 A_{15}
Level —9	—9 A_7, A_8, A_9	—9

Figure 5.4. The presentation of diseases.

(a) A patient with symptoms and behavioral signs only; no lower-level abnormalities are present (e.g., depression, schizophrenia).
(b) An asymptomatic patient with only lower-level abnormalities (e.g., early malignant disease, "chemical diabetes").
(c) A patient having both symptoms and lower-level abnormalities (e.g., thyrotoxicosis, uremia).

By introducing the hierarchical dimension into our disease descriptions, the epistemological status of a disease is made more explicit than it would be with a linear string of disease attributes alone. Behavioral or psychiatric disorders will be characterized by extended strings of attributes, lying for the most part at the top levels, although our knowledge of their causes or their pathogeneses may be slight. Figure 5.4(a) also exemplifies the case of patients whom physicians refer to as having "functional disorders." In contrast, a metabolic disease with fewer attributes distributed over several levels suggests that our knowledge of it may be more coherent, and our understanding a deeper one. Since the attributes that cause a patient to feel ill are clustered among the upper levels, asymptomatic diseases will have only lower level attributes (fig. 5.4b). In the case of the ill *and* diseased individual (fig. 5.4c), the disease attributes occur at both high and low levels, revealing the disease convincingly to both patient and physician.

This model also allows us to emphasize an important distinction in clinical medicine—that between disease and illness. Although these terms are sometimes used interchangeably, it is useful to distinguish between them. One such attempt is that expressed by L. Eisenberg:

> . . . patients suffer illnesses; physicians diagnose and treat "diseases"
> . . . illnesses are *experiences* of disvalued changes in states of being
> . . . diseases, in the scientific paradigm of modern medicine, are *abnormalities* in the *structure* and *function* of body organs and systems. [34]

Illnesses, we might be tempted to say, are "subjective" matters, and diseases are "objective" ones. We can now do better than this and put the issue directly: illnesses are high-level matters and diseases are lower-level ones. When these happen to co-occur, when a patient's "disvalued changes" correspond to a physician's findings of abnormalities in structure or function, the medical-care process can proceed as well as current medical knowledge permits. The occurrence of disease without illness is a situation calling for great tact and skill on the part of a physician, if the patient's interest is to be served. It is with poorly informed or poorly motivated patients that the problem of therapeutic noncompliance lies. The occurrence of illness without disease may be even more troublesome, and this combination raises the greatest difficulties for physicians. Curiously, this does not seem to have been so in the past. Before medical knowledge had reached its current state, and before effective therapy had become widely available, medical treatment was for the most part a high-level enterprise. Being rarely able to treat lower-level causes and dysfunctions, physicians made correspondingly greater efforts to alleviate patients' distress. Because of this, patients could immediately sense that the doctor was trying to help. But medicine's success in discovering lower-level explanations for many illnesses (and providing the opportunity for low-level and specific treatment) seems to make some physicians less understanding with the patients in whom these are not to be found.

As noted before, the conventional explanation of disease processes is asymmetric with respect to level. We can explain (account for) iron deficiency anemia (level —7 of table 5.1) to some degree, in terms of the availability (dietary supply and absorption) of iron (level —9 of table 5.1). We cannot, however, explain a patient's low serum iron by merely saying that he is anemic. We are here using "explanation" in the sense of describing or tracing a causal chain that is believed to underlie a pathogenetic process. Explanation, in this sense, has a direction opposite to that of the flow of causality. And explanation is most frequently sought by examining affairs at lower levels.

Why are lower-level medical explanations so attractive? What makes us believe that if we take things apart we will better understand how they work, and are thus moved to go on and take the parts themselves apart? There is at least one way in which we might attempt to account for this, and it goes to the heart of the scientific method. When we attempt to explain or account for something, we do so by making the fewest assumptions possible. This is the well-known Principle of Parsimony and, being commonly attributed to William of Ockham (or Occam), is referred to as Occam's Razor. The principle asserts that, when faced with alternative explanations, we are safest from error in choosing the one based on the fewest assumptions. When we have a patient with substernal pain radiating to the left arm, diaphoresis, and hypotension, we can account for these findings in at least two ways. Hypotheses (1) myocradial infarction; hypothesis (2) reflux esophagitis, a cervical rib, and acute adrenal failure. These hypotheses are equally logical, but we would not hesitate to choose the former, because it makes fewer assumptions. In the long run we will be correct more often by doing this.

A particular formulation of this principle was made by C. O. Morgan in his study of animal behavior, when he stated, "In no

case may we interpret an action as the outcome of the existence of
a higher psychical faculty, if it can be interpreted as the outcome
of one which stands lower in the psychological scale'' [87]. This is
sometimes known as Morgan's Canon.[8]

We might well explain the abnormal behavior of a patient with
hepatic encephalopathy as being due to possession by demons, as
it probably once was. The difficulty with this is not so much that
demons are hard to demonstrate, but that the explanation is *too
powerful.* By invoking demons we can explain anything, but in so
doing we succeed in explaining nothing. Instead, we would explain
this behavior in terms of elevated blood-ammonia levels or the
like, which accounts for far less (is more parsimonious) and is limited to a few things that we can observe or measure. However, we
cannot get along entirely with lower-level explanations any more
than we can do without multiple causes. But we turn to these alternatives only when the evidence forces us to do so, and even then
we do ''not proliferate causes unnecessarily.''

It is beginning to be more widely recognized that there are
important exceptions to this reductionist practice, and they are
perhaps most obvious in the case of psychosomatic disorders. If
we believe that there are stress-induced diseases, such as peptic
ulcer, we are obliged to regard upward explanation (or downward
causality) as fully as legitimate as the reverse.[9] The reductionist's
method of seeking causes only at lower levels might seem to have
retarded a better understanding of the phenomenon of downward
causation. The importance of the latter has received relatively little
emphasis, despite occasional inquiries undertaken along psychosomatic lines.

Apart from parsimony (and Morgan's Canon), there are other
reasons for favoring the reductionist bias: lower-level attributes
are sharp and distinct, and they may be measured with ever-
increasing sensitivity and convenience with modern laboratory
instruments. Clinical (higher-level) attributes are not only fuzzy
and ambiguous, they are frequently regarded as being somehow
less ''objective,'' and they almost always call for greater skill for
their observation and description. Although it seems to be generally accepted that stress and anxiety can cause or aggravate
sickness, our official models of disease provide an unsuitable
framework for the study of downward causation. An unfortunate
byproduct of this is that so-called holistic views of health and dis-

ease, which should be a part of normal medicine, have increasingly been left for exploitation by cultists, or even by antiscience movements. Many of those holding extreme positions in this direction, while properly stressing the importance of high-level disease processes, tend to disregard all of our knowledge of lower-level phenomena.

Disease attributes need not, of course, be put on an equal footing when it comes to diagnosis. No matter how characteristic a patient's chest pain may seem, repeatedly normal electrocardiograms obtained over a period of several days, and repeated normal serum enzyme determinations, will not permit the diagnosis of myocardial infarction. Disease attributes taken singly have "diagnostic" or "selection" powers that range widely, and in practice *it is frequently the lower-level attributes that provide the strongest evidence for a diagnosis,* because it is here that necessity and contingency are more readily distinguished. Nevertheless, it is the high-level attributes that make patients ill and they are used as the usual starting point for the physician's diagnostic reasoning. And, with some disorders, they are the only known attributes.

Finally, we can use these concepts to clear up another legacy of the nominalist-attribute dichotomy. This is the question of whether something is to be regarded as a "disease" or as a "syndrome." Although neither practicing physicians nor medical researchers lose much sleep over this question, the dispute continues to provide a living for the nosologists. Now that we have contrasted the nominalist and attribute positions in their extreme forms, and have proposed a model for the description of disease, let us see whether this can shed any light on the disease versus syndrome question.

Stedman's Medical Dictionary (23d edition) tells us that "A disease *entity* [is] characterized usually by at least two of these criteria: a recognized etiologic agent (or agents); an identifiable group of signs and symptoms; consistent anatomical alterations." It then defines *syndrome* as "The aggregate of signs and symptoms associated with every morbid process." This definition of disease seems workable because it is loose enough to cover our everyday needs. It emphasizes a recognized etiologic agent (or agents) without requiring it, although other writers have made this a necessary condition. H. P. Himsworth distinguishes between diseases and syndromes in the following way:

> Disease entity implies that any particular illness has a specific cause, a sort of invariable prerequisite for the illness. The syndrome has, as its philosophical basis, not specific disease factors but a chain of physiological processes, interference with which at any point introduces the same impairment of bodily function. The same syndrome may thus arise from many different causes.... It is rarely possible to define a disease precisely but it is always possible to characterize a syndrome.

This quotation is prominently displayed by Robert H. Durham in his *Encyclopedia of Medical Syndromes* [32] as providing a basis for the distinction, although some readers may find it unsatisfying. One might agree that a "particular illness has a specific cause" or, at least that it has specific causes, but it is not clear why one should exempt syndromes from this requirement. Of two patients, one with a "disease" and the other with a "syndrome," it is difficult to accept that causality is operative in one instance and not in the other. Nor does it seem reasonable to invoke "a chain of physiological processes" for syndromes on one hand, and imply some causal discontinuity separating "specific disease factors" from a resulting disease on the other. Finally, if there is any difference between "disease factors" and "impairment(s) of bodily functions," it must be a subtle one. Up to this point there would not seem to be much difference between diseases and syndromes, *except perhaps in the way we view or speak of them.*

Himsworth's last sentence might seem unexceptionable, and appears to suggest a real difference between diseases and syndromes. It does, and this appears to be the only distinction between the two. The distinction, however, is purely definitional, and reflects no difference in the epistemology or biology of either disease or syndrome. Diseases acquire their status through a process of evolution during which they are observed in a multiplicity of patients, their attributes and manifestations are sorted out, clinical-pathological correlations are frequently discovered, some of their mechanisms may become revealed, and their natural histories become clarified. All these factors occur in varying degrees. Some diseases may be characterized clearly (when lower-level attributes are available), and these can be diagnosed with more confidence. This is the case even though they may have many other contingent attributes which some patients will display and others will not. With syndromes, the opposite is the case. Someone (usually the first describer) selects a set of morbid attributes shared by a usually small number of patients, the co-occurrence of which has not been previously recognized. Then *by definition,* a patient having these particular attributes is said to have or exemplify the syndrome. The definition of the syndrome is drawn in terms of *necessary* attributes alone. In an operational sense *diseases are described, syndromes are defined.* But these are procedural matters involved in the process of naming morbid occurrences, and not issues of substance in terms of what we know or can learn about them.

In *Die Klinische Syndrome,* the two twentieth-century nosologists Bernfried Leiber and Gertrud Olberich attempt to distinguish between these two concepts in terms of a model in which suspected symptom complexes pass through a catchment or concentration process (*Nosologische Sammelbecken*) and emerge as diseases. However, the distinguishing features they rely on in separating diseases and syndromes are the etiology and pathogenesis involved. When these are known or definable, and uniform or constant, a disease is implied. When the etiology is unknown, and/or the pathogenesis is not uniform or follows multiple paths, a syndrome is suggested. This distinction, although systematic enough, does not seem to reflect actual medical practice. Rheumatoid arthritis is surely regarded as a disease although both its etiology and pathogenesis are obscure. Banti's Syndrome, in contrast, has a fairly well-defined pathogenesis, and its etiology is better understood.

The suggestion of Leiber and Olberich that when new diseases are first dimly recognized they go through a maturation process as new attributes are found and an improved understanding emerges seems correct. But when a name becomes firmly attached, and the disease can be recognized by observing various combinations of clinical attributes (necessary *or* contingent), it becomes more susceptible to the nominalist's account, and escapes the definitional rigidity of a syndrome. Because a morbid entity can be viewed either as a disease or as a syndrome, depending upon how one chooses to describe or define it, it is not clear that there is any benefit to be gained in maintaining the distinction. Both diseases and syndromes can be equally well represented as networks of clinical attributes, and these then summarize all that we know about them. Beyond this, there is no further reality to be had.

5.5 Disease Classification: The Coding Problem

A long-standing difficulty in medicine has been the lack of a uniform nomenclature for diseases. Medical communications, record keeping, and the computerization of medical information have been plagued by this. Most diseases have more than a single name. Sometimes one of these is the name of the individual who first called it to the attention of the medical world (e.g., Bright's disease, Hodgkin's disease, Parkinson's disease). Occasionally, multiple individuals are so honored (e.g., Laurence-Moon-Biedl syndrome). The modern trend in the naming of diseases has been to abandon the use of such eponyms in favor of names that provide a clue to the pathology involved, for example, glomerulonephritis instead of Bright's disease. There are occasional exceptions to this trend, however, such as the currently increasing use of "Hansen's disease" in place of "leprosy" (presumably because of the adverse public reaction to the latter), and of "Down's syndrome" rather than "mongolism." Some disease names consist of a latinized description of what is directly seen (erythema annulare centrifugum) or otherwise detected (situs inversus viscerum abdominalis). The latter condition is more commonly expressed in its English rendition (transposition of the abdominal viscera), although the former is not. Diseases acquire their names through a variety of different processes, and there is little uniformity as to type or structure.

There is, however, considerable practical importance in the uniform naming of diseases, and the greatest pressure to bring this about has come from public health authorities and epidemiologists. The collecting and processing of public health data require that a single name be consistently applied to a particular set of morbid attributes. As a matter of convenience, it has become customary to assign a second name in the form of a numerical code. The use of a number to stand for a name does not, of course, change the ontology of things in the least. Specifically, it does not by itself introduce any quantitative properties, since these numbers are used for their cardinality and not their ordinality. The use of numerical disease codes proved convenient with earlier punched-card (Hollerith) machinery, and it continues to have the advantage that, in addition to the representation of single meanings, hierarchical relations among diseases can be readily indicated. Thus the *International Classification of Diseases* (ICD) assigns to the ambiguous entity "chronic liver disease and cirrhosis" the code number 571, following which "chronic hepatitis" is assigned 571.4, and a further variant, the still more specific "(chronic) recurrent hepatitis," is designated as 571.49. This approach creates a hierarchical structure and results in the grouping of diseases into classes and subclasses. This procedure also brings related disorders into proximity (biliary cirrhosis, for example, is assigned 571.6), and it provides for the creation of disease categories by means of a range of code numbers (e.g., diseases of the digestive system, in ICD, fall into the range 520-579).

The immediate parent of the disease codes cited in the preceding paragraph is the *International Classification of Diseases,* 9th edition (ICD-9), which was prepared under the auspices of the World Health Organization (WHO) primarily for use in collecting international health statistics. The earlier WHO-produced ICD-8 edition was modified by the U.S. Public Health Service to provide greater detail in certain disease categories, and published for use in the United States as the *International Classification of Diseases—Adapted* (ICDA), 1967. This in turn underwent further revision by the Commission on Professional and Hospital Activities (CPHA) for use in American hospitals for the coding of inpatient medical records, and was published in 1968 as the *Hospital Adaptation of ICDA* (H-ICDA). It will not be our purpose here to review in detail the pedigrees of the disease-coding schemes that have been spawned by the ICD series, which would include, among others, that of the Royal College of General Practitioners, 1972; the International Classification of Health Problems in Primary Care, 1975; the OXMIS Code of the Oxford Community Health Project, 1975; and innumerable local versions produced for use in single institutions.

It is useful to consider this entire family of disease-coding systems in informational terms. These schemes all share one property: if one is provided with the standard name of a disease, it is possible to look up this name in a list and find its unique code number. Synonyms or variant names are also listed and cross-referenced to the standard name, so that if one needed to assign a code to a case of Hennoch-Schoenlein purpura, the cross-reference would lead to "allergic purpura," its standard name, and then to a code number (287.0 in ICD-9-CM). A means is thereby provided for proceeding from an alternative name or synonym to a standard name, and then to a third name, which is a numerical code. For convenience, diseases may be gathered into etiologic categories (e.g., infectious diseases), grouped in terms of the physiological systems affected (e.g., gastrointestinal diseases), or the kind of disease process involved (e.g., neoplastic diseases) or, as ICD does, by using a mixture of all three. These coding schemes, however, deal only with disease names; they lack the capability of either describing a particular instance of disease, or of providing any clinical details about a particular patient. They supply the nominal (together with synonyms for it), but provide no means for representing the attributes of a sick patient. The ICD-derived class of coding methods perpetuate the nominalist view of disease held by its original sponsors and public health officials.

In more recent years, an important step has been taken in disease coding by pathologists who have chosen the opposite approach. The *Systematized Nomenclature of Pathology* (SNOP)[10] consists of a standardized list of terms arranged in the form of a lexicon, in which each term stands for a disease attribute and is assigned a unique code number. These disease attributes are assigned in SNOP to one of four categories (or "axes"): topography —the anatomic site affected; morphology—the structural changes (usually microscopic) associated with the disease; etiology—the cause of the disease; and function—the physiological alterations associated with the disease process. Each attribute appears only once in the lexicon. Terms that can be organized hierarchically (such as anatomic structures) by utilizing their part-whole relations are so grouped. A particular instance of disease (an individual patient's case) can then be described by a series of SNOP code numbers corresponding to the attributes that are observed. SNOP has been widely used, both in the United States and abroad, and it has subsequently undergone important extensions.

In order to increase the range and types of attributes that can be coded, an extended version of SNOP has been developed, which is known as the *Systematized Nomenclature of Medicine* (SNO-MED).[11] The preliminary version of this included two additional attribute categories: "diseases" (which correspond in form to those given in the ICD) and therapeutic "procedures."[12] A still more recent edition has added a third category, or axis, that of "patient occupation." By using all seven categories, a large number of patient attributes can now be numerically coded within the SNOP/SNOMED scheme.

The ICD approach was to introduce a standard nomenclature for the names of diseases and to organize them in a categorical and hierarchical fashion. These diseases were then assigned unique numerical codes for recording them and for reflecting some of the hierarchical relations among them. That resulted in a lexicon of disease names (nominals). The SNOP program was to develop a standardized vocabulary for the recording of disease attributes (the As), and to assign unique numerical codes to these terms. The original ICD and SNOP editions adhered to these respective objectives. Because of increasing pressures to convert health statistics, clinical records, and medical information generally into machine-processible form, the derivatives of these systems now address somewhat mixed goals. The ICD-9-CM edition, for example, provides codes for individuals who, though not ill, may have been exposed to a communicable disease; for those with a past history of a particular disease; and for patients having a family history of some disorder. Codes are also provided for denoting the circumstances under which well individuals seek medical attention, such as for routine physical examinations or for immunizations, or which describe the socioeconomic circumstances of the patient. Still others are available for classifying the events surrounding injuries and poisonings. Nowhere, however, does ICD give the definition or description of any particular disease. In order to define or explain what one is, a complete $(N \parallel A)$ statement must be provided, and ICD lists only the Ns and their synonyms.

The SNOP procedure likewise does not define diseases, since it only provides codes for the As. However, its derivative, SNO-MED, by providing disease names in one of its categories (although not providing the attributes of the cited diseases), supplies standardized lists of both Ns (disease names) and As, which may be assembled by a user to describe a particular *instance of disease*. This is what a patient's medical record does, and the purpose of SNOMED's developers was to provide a means for representing such data in machine-processible form. However, since SNOMED does not provide the information needed to assign disease names to strings of attributes (it would be possible, for example, to code the statement "chicken pox: polyuria, polydipsia, polyphagia") it cannot be said to contain any medical knowledge.

The original employment of the four SNOP categories, or axes, (topography, morphology, etiology, and function) might seem to have been made in an effort to reduce a single lengthy list into four more manageable ones. This division also reflects the kinds of things that pathologists do: the topography section contains the terms needed to describe the gross properties of autopsy or surgical specimens, and the terms needed for describing microscopic observations are included in the section on morphology. Similarly, such disease-causing factors as bacteria, parasites, and toxic substances are included under etiology, and abnormalities of biochemical and physiological processes are described with the terms listed under functions. These four divisions thus closely reflect the pathologists' world of gross and microscopic pathology, microbiology, and clinical pathology. In terms of our hierarchical model, these correspond roughly to four successively lower levels.

The editor of SNOMED added further categories to the four above, which represent a mixture of things so that the desired mutual exclusivity of categories is not always attained. M. Graitson has pointed out the categorical redundancy of morphology and disease—that some situations fit equally well into either, and that the editors have placed "staphylococcal pneumonia" under morphology, whereas "pneumococcal pneumonia" is listed under disease [50]. This redundancy arises because diseases are defined in terms of morphologic (or topographic or functional) primitives. The agenesis of part or all of the upper extremities is, for example, both a topographic description and a disease. These problems are taken care of both in SNOP (where they are less obvious and less common) and in SNOMED by the use of suitable cross-references and pointers. They do not so much detract from the usefulness of these coding methods for their intended purposes as they reflect the difficulty of forming natural classes.

There has been one attempt to introduce a standard nomenclature of disease names that also states what each disease is. This is *Current Medical Information and Terminology* (CMIT), referred to previously.[13] CMIT lists 3,262 diseases arranged alphabetically by preferred name, provides an additional 5,500 or so cross-referenced eponyms and synonyms, and gives the principal clinical, laboratory, X-ray, and pathological attributes that are regarded as being characteristic of each disease. It was not intended to serve as a coding system (although a unique four-digit number is assigned to each disease), and the diseases are listed alphabetically rather than categorically. They are moreover individually assigned to physiological systems, and listed by these systems (in separate tables), so that it provides a rudimentary classification scheme. The text of the book is highly structured, it employs a terse telegraphic style, and each disease definition can be viewed as being in $(N \parallel A)$ form. Since it consists of complete information statements it succeeds in representing a large amount of medical knowledge, and was described by its original editor as a "distillate" of medical knowledge. Although CMIT introduces a standardized vocabulary for disease *names,* it does not attempt to do the same for disease *attributes.* For example, the synonymous terms *pruritus* and *itching* are used interchangeably.

In terms of our information model, there are thus three possible approaches to disease coding and classification:

1. The use of an $(N \parallel -)$ representation, in which the disease names are standardized, linked with synonyms, and assigned numerical codes. By not meeting the completeness condition, this representation can contain no medical information. This is the method employed by the ICD family of codes, and by the earlier (and now largely obsolete) *Standard Nomenclature of Diseases and Operations* (SNDO) [1].

2. The use of the $(- \parallel A)$ representation, in which the disease attributes are given in standard form and assigned numerical codes. This representation, which is also incomplete, cannot contain medical information either. This is the procedure employed by SNOP and its derivatives, SNOMED and SNODERM (*Standard Nomenclature of Dermatology*).

3. The use of the $(N \parallel A)$ representation, in which a complete information statement is provided for each disease, with both the disease name and its attributes being standardized and given numerical codes. This program has been carried out in part by CMIT, in which the disease names are standardized, although the terms used for the attributes are not.

Methods (1) and (2), by not attempting to represent medical knowledge, are in a sense "pure" coding systems. That is, they are standardized nomenclatures that assign code numbers to particular objects—disease names and disease attributes. But according to our hierarchical model, method (1) involves an additional level of abstraction and is, therefore, more sensitive to the state of medical knowledge at a particular time. A disease regarded at one time as a single entity may subsequently be subdivided into several types. If a clinical record lists a disease code that, later on, is replaced by several, there is no way (without having additional information) in which a re-coding of the clinical record can be performed. When, in contrast, disease attributes are coded, there is a better chance that a new disease name can be assigned in the light of newer medical knowledge.

Numerous attempts have been made to introduce structure or standardization into medical records in order to facilitate the filing or retrieval of information. There are probably few physicians who have not at some time attempted a similar procedure with their own office records. Such homemade coding systems are found increasingly in institutions where automated billing systems are used, and they are prevalent where health-services research is actively undertaken. Nearly all these personal or private systems (when they have a coding capability) appear to use method (1). These techniques for representing or classifying diseases have assumed greater importance in recent years as the computer processing of medical information has become feasible, and as the concern with a better understanding of the functioning of the medical-care system grows. The present availability of low-cost microprocessors ("personal computers") has led some physicians to attempt the development of office systems for their own use. This trend will likely add to the pressures for the wider adoption of improved standards for medical record keeping.

5.6 Disease and Health

It has recently become fashionable to speak of "health" rather than "disease," even though we are talking about the same processes or problems. In certain circles, patients are nowadays referred to as "health-care consumers," and physicians and others as "health-care providers." Before adopting such "newspeak," it will be helpful to inquire more closely into what can be meant by "health" and "disease."

The commonsense view of health would seem to be one in which an individual who feels well and who suffers from no disabling bodily or emotional ailments would simply be said to be healthy. This is necessarily a subjective, personal, or psychological view of health. In order to establish this state of affairs we need merely ask someone, "How do you feel?" If we are convinced by the reply "I feel fine," then we would grant (under this psychological view) that the individual is healthy. We must do this even though the individual in question might have asymptomatic hypertension, chemical evidence of early diabetes, or a suspicious shadow on his chest X-ray. In contrast, a physician finding any of these abnormalities (perhaps in the course of a routine examination) would be obliged to inform the patient of such findings and to make suitable recommendations. The physician would do this because he employs a physiological model of health, in which health is defined as the absence of demonstrable disease. It will be noted, however, that in both the private (psychological) and the public (physiological) concepts of health, health is defined by the *absence* of certain kinds of attributes.

This state of affairs leads to an apparent paradox: that disease is somehow a simpler matter to describe or talk about than health. The use of the information model, however, shows that there is no paradox here. To be able to recognize or confirm the occurrence of a disease, we may require knowledge of only a few relevant clinical attributes. It seems likely, for example, that we could distinguish among all the diseases listed in CMIT by means of a dozen or so attributes, and that if we were always to have low-level attributes available to us it might require even fewer. But if we are to affirm that an individual is "healthy," under the physiological view of health, we would need to confirm the absence of thousands of disease attributes. To do this would require that we ask an unimaginably large number of questions about the occurrence of symptoms, search for the presence of all the known physical signs of disease, and perform enormous numbers of laboratory tests. If we were to attempt such an undertaking, and all the results were (miraculously) found to be "normal," we could still only report that the patient was presumably healthy, since the clinical descriptions of human beings are open ones, and we cannot even test for the integrity of all the physiological functions we know about. Moreover, it is clear that no one could possibly pass such a battery of tests since the definition of a "normal" test result is a statistical one having the property that the likelihood of a normal individual giving *only* normal results asymptotically approaches zero as the number of tests increases. In short, there can be no such thing as a "clean bill of health." Under the physiological model, the affirmation of health is an inductive procedure (and hence vulnerable to the results of future observation), whereas the confirmation of disease is a deductive one and can be made with certainty.

Now all this may seem extreme, since these issues do not seem to present great difficulties for medicine, even though some patients will continue to drop dead shortly after "passing" a routine physical examination. Yet physicians are able to perform useful physical examinations of well individuals by ruling out the likelihood of certain common diseases that might be present in asymptomatic form. This kind of examination is worth making because of the value of the early detection of diseases such as hypertension or diabetes, and the consequent ability of the physician to influence their course. So such relatively common diseases will be looked for. Even uncommon diseases may be sought, particularly if they are serious ones, and if suitable (inexpensive and safe) diagnostic procedures are available. Nevertheless, an individual's being healthy (under the physiological view) can never be proven because induction is involved, whereas the affirmation of an existing disease (being deductive) can readily be carried out. This phenomenon, which follows directly from informational considerations, may not make a great deal of difference in the everyday practice of medicine, but it greatly affects how we think about health and disease.

These ideas of what is meant by "disease," and the methods available to us for describing and representing them, will now be used to analyze the processes we employ in obtaining and utilizing clinical information. From the viewpoint of medical information processing, none of these activities is more central to medicine than the matter of diagnosis. This we shall consider next.

6

The Processes of Diagnosis

6.1 The Context of Diagnosis

When used as a noun, "diagnosis" is the result of the naming process, which we considered earlier. This labeling achieves a useful synoptic end by permitting us to summarize a patient's multiple abnormalities with a single word. Used as a verb, "diagnosis" stands for a collection of different perceptual and cognitive acts, including recognition and inference. What these acts are and how they relate to one another are subjects of great interest and importance in medicine. They are sometimes discussed under such headings as "problem solving," "decision making," or "pattern recognition," although it is seldom clear where one of these begins and another ends.

The use of the term *diagnosis* in medicine embraces a range of methods including the direct recognition of some disorders (e.g., acne, psoriasis), the inferring of others from the evidence provided by causal cues (e.g., the occurrence of an instance of a disease during an epidemic of the disease), and a process of hypothesis formation and verification, which is perhaps the most general diagnostic method. The studies of Arthur Elstein and his associates confirm that during diagnosis physicians employ a number of different strategies, and that they do this subconsciously and with great flexibility [35].

Given the variety in the states of affairs that count as disease and the rich repertoire of cognitive methods employed by physicians as they detect, describe, and classify diseases, it would be surprising to discover that some single and unvarying process was employed. Since no such process has been identified, diagnostic skills continue to be taught by example, and the teaching is usually aimed at avoiding certain well-recognized sources of error. One error is to simply overlook a particular possibility; another is to overemphasize the importance of one abnormal finding at the expense of another (misweighting attributes) so that the more important one may fade from consideration. In an attempt to avoid this, diagnosis is sometimes taught as a two-step process: data collection, followed by data interpretation or inference. Medical students are commonly urged to defer making diagnostic hypotheses until the initial data collection (history-taking and physical examination) is completed. Some writers have stressed the organization and formatting of the clinical findings obtained during this phase [134]. However, the deferral of hypothesis-making is rarely, if ever, practiced by physicians [35]. Physicians tend to generate hypotheses early and it is probable that there is never a time during the diagnostic process when the physician does not have one or more candidate diagnoses in mind. Indeed, as we saw in chapter 1 and as Popper has repeatedly stressed, observation itself cannot be carried out without some underlying hypothesis or theory [100]. Observation is "theory-laden," and cannot be carried out unless one is looking for something. Early hypothesis formation is therefore necessary if medical knowledge is to be brought to bear in guiding the clinical investigation of a patient. The trick is not to become wedded to these early hypotheses but to keep an open mind until all the evidence is in. Most important, the diagnostician must at every stage of the process be willing to begin over again. The goal of the diagnostic process is to arrive at a description of the patient's condition that best accounts for all the evidence. Utilizing Occam's Razor, the description the physician ordinarily seeks is the name of a single disease.

It is usually possible, *given a sufficiently extended period of observation,* to decide whether a given diagnosis is correct, although this is not always the case. Some patients will seek medical attention for minor, self-limiting conditions undergoing resolution in which the characteristic symptoms or signs have already disappeared. Others will present their physicians with vague complaints that wax and wane, producing shifting patterns that provide no certain grip. In still other instances, an illness may be misdiagnosed initially but, if the disease is a progressive one, will eventually declare itself. Although certainty is only occasionally available to physicians (either in the clinical data or in the conclusions that can be drawn from them), the goal of the diagnostic process is to achieve the most convincing explanation of the clinical findings in the light of existing knowledge. This goal, however, does not stand as an abstract ideal to be pursued through thick and thin, and at all costs. Diagnoses are made, or attempted, when it is important to have them. But there is always a more important purpose to be served—the patient's own best interests. This is in no way to suggest that these are not generally served by obtaining the "correct" diagnosis. Far from it. But the process of acquiring clinical data will always exact a price in risk, pain, money, or time. In every decision made to acquire additional data, the costs of doing so must be compared with the expected value (to the patient) of the results. Since no patient can ever be studied completely, the diagnostic process has no formal end point. It is here, it is sometimes suggested, that the art of medicine and the science of medicine begin to part company. A line of argument that has been used in this respect is that medicine is value-laden, whereas science is neutral or value-free.[1] It is unnecessary to invoke this argument if diagnosis is properly placed in the context of the medical-care process; that it is always a means and not an end. Thus, although the diagnostic process aspires toward correctness, its methods are tempered by what is appropriate under the circumstances. Diagnosis is part of a continuous and undivided process of medical care, not a prelude to it, or a detached intellectual exercise for which one is to be scored "right" or "wrong." To use the language of gaming, diagnostic success is not judged by the number of games won but by the stakes that are won. Thus the choice of a diagnosis, when treatment is to be chosen, will be influenced by considerations other than the desire to be correct.[2]

The process of diagnosis involves selecting from a list of diseases the single disease that best accounts for the appearance in a patient of a collection of findings, which is always incomplete, and in which the process of observation itself is constrained by medical, ethical, and economic factors. It is necessary to be mindful of the complexity of this overall process when we turn to specific abstractions in which many of these details become lost.

6.2 Diagnosis As Recognition

Some diagnoses can be made at a glance. One looks at a patient, and a name comes to mind. We recognize a friend, our car, or our overcoat in much the same way. And just as it sometimes happens with our friends, our car, or our overcoat, we occasionally make mistakes. Seen at a distance or under poor lighting, what we judge to be an acquaintance will turn out to be a stranger. Or we may find ourselves attempting to unlock another's car, if it happens to resemble our own. We are impressed by such cases of misrecognition because recognition itself is so rapid, reliable, and taken for granted. The failure to recognize a familiar disease becomes more likely when a case presents in an unusual manner, or differs in significant respects from the exemplar of its class. Diagnosis by recognition occurs most commonly through visual perception, *prima vista,* and particularly in such specialties as dermatology, radiology, and pathology, where the disease includes many morphological attributes.

When we recognize such diseases as psoriasis or vitiligo, we do so by apprehending the disease in its totality. We do not stop to analyze the individual features; at least not until the diagnosis has been made presumptively and we are attempting to confirm it. With other modes of diagnosis, we perform various kinds of abstractions first, isolating individual features and considering them in various combinations. When we recognize diseases, however, we do not do this, any more than we recognize a familiar face by first analyzing its individual features.

After a medical student has seen half a dozen cases of untreated psoriasis in the clinic, he or she would be able to recognize this disease accurately in a typical established case. After three years of training, a dermatology resident will recognize uncommon variants of this disorder; cases presenting with a few pustules or with an itching erythema of the palms, with only dandruff and itching of the scalp, or perhaps with fingernail deformities. This type of diagnosis does not seem to be made by any process of deductive or causal reasoning—there is very little to reason from. The thing seen is the disease, not causes for it. There is no causative agent that one knows, no laboratory test gives a clue, and the symptoms are few. One simply looks at a lesion and, if one knows the disease, one recognizes it. This kind of recognition occurs when we see a patient with acne or vitiligo, or as we watch the gait of a patient with Parkinson's disease, or tabes dorsalis. Once recognition has begun, it subconsciously draws our attention to other features in our search for supporting evidence. Seeing psoriatic lesions on the backs of a patient's hands, we glance at the nails; noting the shuffle of a person with Parkinson's disease, we may look for the characteristic facial appearance.

There are many diseases and conditions that are recognized by simply observing physical lesions or noting the alterations of normal functions. In such instances, the disease itself is directly seen. Recognition also occurs through our other senses—trained ears will detect (with the stethoscope) the murmurs of aortic insufficiency or mitral stenosis, and skilled touch will reveal hidden masses in locations where none should be.

"Recognition" is sometimes extended to a broader collection of percepts. R. L. Engle writes, "Diagnosis may be defined as the art, science, or act of recognizing disease from signs, symptoms, or laboratory data" [36]. Compared with the direct recognition of diseases, this extension to such intangible things as symptoms and laboratory data may seem curious, since patient complaints and test results may have referents that cannot be directly apprehended by our senses. Recognition thus has a peculiar status, and it has been regarded by psychologists as lying somewhere between perception and cognition [83]. If it is appropriate to extend recognition to include things that are not directly perceived, there seems little reason not to accept that our encountering the words *polyphagia, polydipsia,* and *polyuria* leads to the recognition of the disease diabetes mellitus. Because of examples such as these the diagnostic process has been considered by some physicians to be predominantly an act of recognition. This is sometimes spoken of as "pattern recognition," and posits that instances of disease are characterized by recurring and conjoined attributes, which are directly recognized as such. There can be no dispute with the suggestion that *some* diseases are, in fact, diagnosed in this manner, and several have already been mentioned which fit this model. What remains to be seen is whether this model of the human diagnostic process can be usefully generalized.

The pattern recognition model of diagnosis has received much attention in recent years because it is one that in favorable cases can be abstracted and represented mathematically, and therefore carried out with a computer. Such computer programs have sometimes produced remarkable results, and they have become interesting objects of study in their own right. A question which we will consider here is whether such programs are to be taken as models of human diagnostic performance. In considering diagnostic computer programs, it is useful to distinguish between the view that the operation of the program reproduces in some significant way a process employed by the human diagnostician, or whether it is a mechanical (formal) way of arriving at a diagnosis by independent (nonhuman) methods. The difference between these two views is not always made clear by writers on this subject, and the existence of such a distinction has even been denied [77].

In their influential paper on medical reasoning, Robert Ledley and Lee Lusted state at the outset: "Before computers can be used effectively for (diagnostic) purposes, however, we need to know more about how the physician makes a medical diagnosis" [66]. There seems little doubt that such knowledge would be helpful if it were available, but is it really necessary? This strategy, in which one first attempts to discover how some natural (frequently, biological) process is carried out, and then constructs a machine to imitate it, has for long had a certain commonsense appeal. The principal difficulty with it is that it does not appear to provide a method of general usefulness. The wheel, for example, has made a vastly greater contribution to methods of ground transportation than have efforts to imitate mechanically the actions of legs and feet. Neither do successful machine tools nor automatic dishwashers in any way simulate the action of hands or arms. The imitation of bird flight, as a precursor activity to the development of the airplane, seems to have made relatively minor contributions. It was by abandoning efforts to construct machines with flapping wings (i.e., attempts to attain both aerodynamic support and propulsion with a single mechanism) that practical heavier-than-air flight was achieved. Success came when aircraft designers stopped trying to imitate birds, and learned more about fluid dynamics and propulsion, subjects presumably unknown to birds. In short, our technology seems to make the most rapid progress by aiming directly at useful goals, rather than by adopting the diversionary course of first attempting to understand how people or animals may achieve the same ends.

A secondary reward sometimes attributed to the simulation

approach is that, if one attains by means of a machine some end that is naturally achieved by human beings, it will contribute to an understanding of human performance. This is the previous line of argument in reverse, and it seems at best questionable. Finally, one would surely suppose that both goals could not be sought at the same time; that one could not design a machine to *simulate* human performance and at the same time claim that the same machine helps *explain* human performance. But there have been instances in which something very much like this has happened.

There are troubles enough when either of these goals is sought alone. We read, for example, "An equation of conditional probability is derived to express the logical process used by a clinician in making a diagnosis from clinical data" [132]. The equation mentioned was shown to be as accurate in diagnosing as three experienced cardiologists using the same clinical data in an experiment with thirty-six cases among which there were thirty-two possible congenital heart conditions. But this is neither a demonstration that the cardiologists employed this equation (it is unlikely that they had ever heard of it) nor that the equation itself modeled or simulated whatever processes the cardiologists used (these being unknown). The result of this experiment permits one to conclude simply that an explicit mathematical method worked as well as the unknown means of reasoning employed by the physicians. But the fact that two processes produce similar results is the weakest of evidence that the processes themselves are alike. A similarity in outcome can at most raise the possibility that the processes *might* be alike. This particular diagnostic problem was a well-structured one which, the authors showed, was capable of being reduced to a computation. The cardiologists could just as well have used pencil and paper and performed the computation, if the formula and the relevant conditional probabilities had been known to them.[3] If a clinical problem has a single, clear, and definite method of solution and a "correct" answer, a computational procedure cannot be outperformed by methods based upon informal or heuristic reasoning.

This is not to imply that computers cannot be used in appropriate cases for the performance of tasks in ways roughly similar to the ways in which human beings perform them. In highly abstract applications such as process control and bookkeeping, the flow sheets reflect the fact that some complex operations can be decomposed into simpler ones, and that among these simpler ones there may be well-structured problems having algorithmic solutions. If this were not the case we could not have industrial production machinery. It is in the possibility of identifying just such problems that much of the promise of computers in medicine lies.

Direct and immediate recognition by the physician appears sufficient to account for the entire diagnostic process with the kinds of diseases already mentioned, and it is probably involved with others. Bolinger and Ahlers [17], taking a Shannon theory view of diagnosis, have estimated the reduction in diagnostic uncertainty at different stages of the diagnostic process. They report that the average uncertainty was reduced by two-thirds during initial face-to-face contacts with patients who eventually were found to have a single disease. They conclude that the striking reduction in uncertainty achieved during the initial contacts with patients, and during the early formulation of complaints (but prior to a complete history) could only have occurred by a process of pattern recognition.

Although some diseases or disease categories may be immediately recognized at this early point, it seems equally probable that this portion of the patient-physician encounter is concerned with a rapid and approximate diagnostic scanning. This time may be spent in the identification of relevant attributes, and in the creation of high-level diagnostic categories and hypotheses. Much of this "reasoning" may be carried out subconsciously, it may well involve parallel processing, and it is frequently difficult or impossible to later recall exactly what occurred. The information acquired during this initial contact with a patient is also influenced by the context (cultural, environmental, and so forth), and much of this information is implicitly included or excluded. The work reported by Bolinger and Ahlers was carried out in the *medical ward* of a teaching hospital where a large number of potential diagnoses would have been subconsciously dismissed even *before* the patient was seen—for example, obstetric, pediatric, and many surgical diseases would not likely have come under consideration. The first glimpse of the patient affords a further partitioning in the set of possible diagnoses. If the patient is seen to be male, gynecological diseases are eliminated. If the patient is resting comfortably, entire categories of medical emergencies can be set aside. Large amounts of nonverbal information are acquired very rapidly by physicians, and in this whole matter of establishing context most of what goes on does so subconsciously. The authors' conclusion that the information obtained in the very earliest contact with the patient greatly reduced the diagnostic uncertainty is entirely in accord with the experience of most physicians.

A similar investigation was conducted with patients referred to a medical outpatient clinic in Great Britain. The study was conducted prospectively, and the examining physician's current clinical diagnosis (together with an associated confidence factor) was recorded following each step of the examination. For more than half of the patients seen the diagnosis was changed from that originally proposed by the referring practitioner after the patients had been studied in the clinic. Of those cases in which a change of diagnosis was made at some point in the consultation, more than two-thirds were made following the history-taking alone. The physical examination and laboratory testing were responsible for about 15 percent each [54].

Whether the large amount of clinical data acquired in the earliest portion of the workup occurs through some single kind of cognitive act, which would justify our calling it pattern recognition, or whether the clues obtained support the formation of higher-level hypotheses, which may serve as diagnostic way stations (e.g., such concepts as "infectious disease," "surgical abdomen") remains to be seen. But apart from specific diseases that are diagnosed by being directly seen, it seems likely that experienced clinicians employ a similar technique with nonvisual disease attributes, among which they search for a sense of pattern or structure. This kind of diagnosis occurs as the recognition of something already known [31].

6.3 Diagnosis As Classification

Although the recognition model can account for the diagnostic process in many cases, it cannot serve as a general diagnostic method. For one thing, it seems excessively dependent on the existence of archetypical patterns or exemplars of diseases. Such devices are useful for teaching medical students, and they are no doubt employed to some degree by all physicians. But diagnosis frequently involves more than recognition. It is not the typical or readily recognized cases that cause difficulties in diagnosis. It is the cases that do not closely match the exemplars or those that present with atypical features that do. Recognition will not help here and we need different methods to deal with these cases. The procedure we shall examine next is that of *classification*. When we classify things, we no longer deal with an object in its totality but with its attributes individually. Classification is concerned with attributes, and in order to isolate these we need first an appropriate abstraction of the whole object.

We have considered some features of "similarity" (in section 4.3), but the notion of classification as it relates to diagnosis has not yet been examined. We now have the tools, so it is appropriate to do so now. Much of the recent activity in the theory of classification has occurred in biology, and this interest has been intensified by the availability of the computer.

The word *classification* is used both to describe the process of assigning objects to classes (that is, of identifying them) and to refer to the process of constructing systems of classes and categories which permit this. The attributes of objects differ in kind and quality, and they serve different purposes when it comes to classification. If some feature of an object is accidental or contingent it can tell us little about the object. A necessary attribute, however, establishes an object's eligibility or raises the possibility of its belonging to a particular class. And, finally, the possession of a sufficient attribute will guarantee membership of an object in the class. The role of these different kinds of attributes in the process of classification will be better seen as we examine two contrasting approaches to taxonomy.

One is known as the *monothetic* method. Monothetic classifications are those in which the conditions for class membership differ by at least one property (attribute) from nonmembership, and this property is uniformly possessed by all members of the class [17]. For example, in the universe of polygons, the class of triangles consists of figures that have three sides. This single feature distinguishes absolutely between membership and nonmembership in the class of triangles. This key property upon which classification depends is, in this instance, both necessary *and* sufficient. This method of classifying works in both directions: an object possessing this property is necessarily a member of the class, and an object not having it cannot be a member. This method is therefore a particularly incisive one, but it turns out to be useful only with relatively simple objects. The monothetic method is not of general usefulness to us in medicine nor with high-level objects because of the difficulty in establishing the necessity and sufficiency of attributes. It is a highly specialized matter, for example, to find a single such property that makes a dog a dog, and which at the same time is possessed by no other animal. Yet it is easy to find the key property for triangles.

An alternative approach has therefore been proposed in an attempt to avoid the Aristotelian essentialism inherent in the monothetic procedure. This approach is termed the *polythetic*. It rejects the notion that any one attribute is more significant than any other, and assigns equal importance to all of them.[4] In practice, this method requires that a large number of attributes be determined before classification can proceed. Since no single attribute is accorded preeminence over any other, the similarity of different objects is measured entirely in terms of the *number* of shared attributes. This gives to the procedure a thoroughgoing statistical flavor, and it has become referred to as *numerical taxonomy*. The attractiveness of the polythetic approach arises from its algorithmic nature, and from the power of the computer for classifying when this is combined with statistical tools, such as clustering procedures. Above all, this method might appear to sidestep the thorny issue of having to decide what is essential or relevant. Among the advocates of this approach, P. H. A. Sneath has argued that the classifications derived in this way are "natural" classifications [120].

Yet one may wonder whether natural categories are likely to be generated by a procedure that treats all attributes of an object as being of equal significance because of our ignorance of a subject. Moreover, the procedure ignores our partial knowledge of the laws of nature as these are expressed in the relationships among attributes. Reasoning that ignores not only relevance (on the grounds that we have no basis for determining it) but natural laws as well might seem to reject too much. It would seem analogous to an argument that two circles slightly different in size are really *very much unlike,* because they differ in so many different respects, that is, in radius, in diameter, in circumference, and in area. When the underlying laws or connections among things are ignored, attributes can be identified and enumerated at great length without increasing understanding. Other criticisms have been made of numerical taxonomy; some of these have been pointed out by Vernon Pratt, with the arguments:

> ...there is no such number as the number of characters an individual organism can be said to have, and so no sense in saying that a certain organism has more characters in common with a second than it does with a third. First it is easy to see that even if you can begin to count the number of characters possessed by an organism, you could never complete the job; but second...it is a job one cannot in reality even begin. ("Numerical Taxonomy—A Critique," *Jour. Theor. Biol.* [1972], 36: 581-592)

The first of Pratt's criticisms is consistent with the idea of an open information statement being the form in which natural objects are necessarily described. His second point is that the number of characters is description-relative and that, unless a description is first specified, the characters cannot be counted at all.

Other reservations about the polythetic assumption that all attributes of an object are to be taken as being on an equal footing arise for a different reason. If the relevance of attributes counted for nothing in classification (which is the proposition entailed by the concept of uniform weighting), any effort to produce a more accurate description of an object by the careful choice of attributes would be doomed to failure. But this would also follow for intentional attempts to produce a *less* accurate description. From this it would seem that all descriptions of equal length must be of equal quality. This hardly seems consistent with our knowledge of the quality of clinical descriptions.

How is it possible that numerical taxonomy appears to succeed so well in practice in the hands of bacteriologists and botanists if this procedure is subject to the above criticisms? The answer seems to lie in the circumstance that by considering objects that lie at the same hierarchical level, and by employing attributes that are frequently biochemical, they are using many necessary attributes. S. P. Lapage and others have described how they went about choosing the attributes of bacteria to be used in applying this method: "A range of tests was selected which included tests for as many different enzymes and biochemical pathways as possible, e.g., the electron transport system and those involved in the metabolism of carbon and nitrogen compounds" [65]. These authors themselves do not assert the extreme form (uniform weighting) of numerical taxonomy but instead view the classification process as one dealing with the conditional probabilities of attributes. That is, they concede the need for weighting attributes. Their procedure for selecting attributes, however, would seem almost to guarantee that many of them will be necessary ones and, with necessary attributes in hand, the issue of relevancy has already been bypassed. As Robert Sokal has remarked, the useful classifications, which are based upon *a few attributes,* are usually to be found in the physical sciences where they reflect some underlying law [121]. But it is precisely the effect of underlying laws which makes some attributes relevant and others not. This is what natural laws are about. And there are laws and regularities in biochemistry also, so that by choosing attributes that reflect the rules of biochemistry one is more likely to be selecting necessary than contingent ones. It seems that the polythetic procedure works well in bacteriology because bacteriologists employ low-level attributes. The attributes most likely to be chosen, even if they were to be selected at random, stand a good chance of being necessary ones so that relevancy is assured.

But this local success, occurring for clear and understandable reasons, need not guarantee that the method will be equally successful when applied to the classification of higher-level objects. There is little doubt that, even if rather casual observations of natural objects are processed by means of clustering procedures, evidence of structure will be obtained. But the structure that is revealed may not be what is sought, because the solutions are underdetermined until we set limits upon the kinds of answers in which we are interested. And what we mean by "being interested in" is again nothing other than this matter of relevancy.

From our previous considerations of fuzziness and ambiguity as they arise in hierarchical systems, we can now see how certain specific issues in classification might be approached. For atoms and molecules, classification raises few uncertainties; necessity and contingency can be readily told apart, and sufficient attributes are found in abundance. Knowing its optical emission spectrum is sufficient for the correct identification of any chemical element. There is no further Aristotelian "essence" to be sought. When we deal with more complex objects, such as living things, we find that large numbers of emergent attributes have come into existence. These natural properties are continually being discovered as our knowledge of biology and medicine increases. And as this knowledge grows and becomes more detailed, the necessary attributes of particular things become clearer to us. When we employ these necessary attributes in our descriptions, our classification methods can be revised and made more effective. Diseases that were formerly lumped together as a single entity become distinguishable on the basis of newer knowledge. But in order to perform this separation, we must first decide which attributes are characteristic of one disease and not another. It is only when we have done this that we can say that we have knowledge of these diseases.

In light of these considerations, it is useful to think of diagnosis in terms of classification and as involving estimates of similarity— an alternative process to the direct recognition of diseases. This notion becomes particularly attractive when we recall that a disease definition is a class definition. This is clear when we remember how textbook descriptions of disease are formulated in the first place. Well-defined diseases are just those that are capable of being described in detail. These written descriptions of disease are also cumulative ones, in that some of the attributes noted in one patient are combined with other attributes observed in other patients having the same disease. No patients with a particular disease will display all the attributes which the textbooks associate with it. This process results in the conventional (textbook) descriptions of disease arising in the following way. Patient 1, having a particular disease, is noted to have attributes $A_1, A_3, A_6, A_8, A_{10}, A_{11}$, and Patient 2 (having what is considered to be the same disease[5]) is described as having $A_1, A_3, A_8, A_{10}, A_{11}$. As additional patients are studied, further information is collected, and *the attributes originally predicated of individual patients finally become attributed to the disease itself.* That is, a shift from the attribute to the nominalist view of disease has occurred. Then one can combine the descriptions obtained from a large number of individual patients:

$$(D \parallel A_1 \; A_3 \qquad A_6 \qquad\quad A_{10} \; A_{11}) \qquad \text{from Patient 1}$$
$$(D \parallel A_1 \; A_3 \qquad\qquad\quad A_8 \; A_{10} \; A_{11}) \qquad \text{from Patient 2}$$

$$\vdots$$

$$(D \parallel A_1 \qquad A_4 \qquad\qquad A_{10} \; A_{11}) \qquad \text{from Patient n}$$

Our textbook description of D will eventually come to read something like "Patients with D will always display (or have) A_1, A_{10}, and A_{11}, they will frequently have A_3, and they may have A_4, A_6, and A_8."[6]

Let us say that in the previous schema D is myocardial infarction, A_1 is chest pain, A_{10} is an ECG showing an appropriate type of abnormality, and A_{11} is pathologically confirmed myocardial necrosis. If A_{11} were chosen as the defining attribute of the disease the diagnosis of D could not be made in a living patient. If, however, A_{10} were chosen to be the defining attribute (which is reasonable if we have evidence that A_{10} and A_{11} always co-occur) the diagnosis of D could be made in living patients. This, of course, is what is done. But many individuals suddenly die, having had symptoms of chest pain radiating to the arm (A_3), nausea (A_4), cold sweating (A_6), and shock (A_8), for whom neither an ECG was obtained prior to death nor an autopsy performed after death. Such patients will still have "myocardial infarction" recorded on their death certificates as the cause of death, a polythetic diagnosis.

We can and do make medical diagnoses, as well as psychiatric ones, on the basis of contingent attributes alone. The polythetic procedure can indeed be made to work, and it may be all that we have. Until the discovery of the LE cell test by M. M. Hargraves [7], the necessary attributes of systemic lupus erythematosus were only those to be found at autopsy. Yet this disorder was frequently diagnosed during life, in the 1930s and 1940s, on the basis of high-level and contingent attributes alone. Making a diagnosis does not require that we find the patient to have an attribute that is a necessary one for the disease in question (let alone a sufficient one), although the failure to do so will reduce the degree of confidence associated with the diagnosis.

If it can be established that a necessary attribute is absent in a particular patient, the corresponding disease can be rejected on the basis of this single finding alone. That is why the "ruling out" of diseases is such a powerful procedure in diagnosis. It is a purely deductive procedure with respect to the hypothesis in question, and can lead to a certain conclusion. The confirmability of absent attributes may, of course, present serious practical problems. One of these is the matter of sampling. A needle biopsy specimen of the liver that is found not to contain tumor, cannot be interpreted to exclude hepatic metastases, nor do the results of a nerve biopsy which are negative for acid fast organisms exclude leprosy. However, repeatedly normal blood pressure measurements would exclude the diagnosis of hypertension. And if hypertension is a necessary attribute of some other disorder it would exclude that as well. Another problem is that of test sensitivity and specificity. X-ray examinations, isotopic scans, and ultrasound studies, for example, all have their characteristic thresholds of sensitivity (detectability) for particular abnormalities. Lesions below some threshold size will always escape detection, and the report of a normal examination is always interpreted in this light. The usefulness of a laboratory test is greatest when the attribute being measured is necessary, and the specificity is highest if the attribute happens to be pathognomonic (sufficient), or has a high conditional probability for a given disease.

It would seem that neither the pure monothetic nor the polythetic programs can be taken to model the process of diagnosis by classification. To assume that the monothetic will always succeed is to assume that we always have necessary (or, better, sufficient) attributes available to us and that in a sense we know almost everything. In medicine this assumption is simply unwarranted. Monothetic diagnosis in medicine is effective in instances in which we know a great deal about a disease, and in particular when we have specific (sufficient) attributes available. Diseases involving a specific enzyme deficiency are a good example. When this knowledge is unavailable to us, and particularly when the only clinical attributes known are high-level ones, we must use the polythetic method. This requires that we have a larger number of abnormalities in hand, and that we have a suitable strategy for making inferences from them. But when the polythetic method, which insists upon the equal weighting of attributes and dismisses relevance and necessity, assumes that we know almost nothing about a disease, it ignores too much. Medical knowledge is only occasionally in such a bleak state.

Diagnosis in practice (to the extent that it follows the classification model) usually falls in between these monothetic and polythetic extremes. The diagnostician places a high premium upon the necessary attributes of disease. Laboratory medicine and specific testing methods have therefore played an increasingly dominant role in diagnosis in recent years. If laboratory testing is overused, as some analysts of the medical-care process suggest, this would seem to result in large part from the physician's intuition that it is at these lower descriptive levels that the necessary and sufficient attributes of disease are most likely to be found.

We must also ask whether a finding which may be necessary to the diagnosis of a particular disease need be specific to it. That is, can two or more different diseases have the same necessary attributes? The answer, of course, is that they can. Necessity and sufficiency are different kinds of things. Fever and leukocytosis are necessary attributes, for all practical purposes, for entire categories of infectious diseases. Conversely, a finding such as Koplik spots, which is considered to be pathognomonic and sufficient, need not be necessary. Since, apart from the defining attribute(s), all other attributes of diseases are contingent, we would like to know something of their relative importance or frequency. This information, unfortunately, is rarely available, except as reflected in the personal experience of physicians. We do not yet have the comprehensive and systematic data that will allow us to answer the following questions. If a patient has disease D_1, what is the probability that attribute A_1 will be present; that is, $P(A_1 \mid D_1)$? If a patient has A_1, what is the probability that D_1 is the correct diagnosis; that is, $P(D_1 \mid A_1)$? The uses to which such data could be put, possible means for collecting them, and some of the limitations in their use will be considered later.

Diagnosis can be viewed under the classification model as a process for comparing the attributes of a particular patient with the attributes of a particular disease definition, and applying a measure by means of which we can express the degree of similarity between the two. Having done this, we may repeat the process with a second disease, a third, and so on. We can then select the diseases that most clearly resemble the patient's, discard those that seem unlikely, and create a differential diagnosis. This is the list of candidate diagnoses that best fit what is known about the patient at a given stage of the diagnostic process. This process can then be continued. As additional clinical attributes become known, this differential diagnosis will change. Newly found attributes may be incompatible with a disease on the list, permitting us to reject it, or they may add further diseases to the list. The process of diagnosis, however, is only in part a sequential one, and it is never irreversible. Upon receipt of new and conflicting data, the physician will quickly return to earlier stages of the inference process.

6.4 Diagnostic Reasoning and Causality

Of the several modes of reasoning that may be employed in diagnosis, one of the more easily recognized and recounted is analysis based upon causality.[7] Confronted with a particular clinical finding, and with his attention focused upon it, the physician may automatically seek a cause for it. When such a cause is being sought, it will be its general fitness and its ability to explain other clinical findings that will determine its value. A hypothetical cause with a high explanatory value will prevail over one that accounts for less, and the nature of this "explanation," or "accounting for," is fundamental to this kind of reasoning.

The process resulting from this instinctive desire to explain matters results in a quite different type of diagnostic goal. Instead of having a disease name as its immediate objective, or merely the listing of abnormalities found in a patient, it will seek causes for specific abnormalities and connections among them. Unlike the preceding types of diagnosis, this striving for a causal explanation depends on the biological knowledge of how things work. Since medicine deals with a uniquely complex natural object, the network of possibilities that underlies medical explanations is a particularly rich one. This leads to a situation in medicine that may set a trap for the physician, a situation that is not always kept in mind. As the number of possible causes for a state of affairs becomes greater, the ease of finding a plausible explanation will increase as well. During the process of diagnosis, the correct answer is always *underdetermined* until the very end. That is, several different diagnoses or explanations may have equal force, given the clinical information available at the time. J. R. Platt has humorously illustrated how this works in a different context.

> Some cynics tell a story, which may be apocryphal, about the theoretical chemist who explained to his class, "And thus we see that the C-Cl bond is longer in the first compound than in the second because the percent of ionic character is smaller." A voice from the back of the room said, "But Professor X, according to the Table, the C-Cl bond is shorter in the first compound." "Oh, is it?," said the professor, "Well, that's still easy to understand, because the double-bond character is higher in that compound." [96]

The translation of this anecdote into a medical example can readily be done by any physician.

An influence which tends to act in concert with the too-ready explanation is the understandable need in medicine to have a rational basis for any selected course of action. Few physicians would feel comfortable in making a diagnosis that did not have a convincing appeal to them, or in employing a treatment that had neither a rational basis of action nor a credible claim of efficacy. However, the opportunities for finding support for a particular diagnostic or therapeutic choice are great within the body of today's medical knowledge. When we have only partial information we may argue either side of some proposition with equal effectiveness. Arguments based upon plausibility, or upon what may be possible rather than upon certain knowledge, are highly seductive and correspondingly risky. Yet if we were always to insist upon certainty, we would accomplish very little. And if we were to withhold treatment that was known to be effective because we did not understand (to the last detail) how it worked, medical practice would be little advanced beyond that of the Middle Ages.

To put this in perspective, consider the differences in the structure of, say, medical knowledge or human biology and that of, say, electrical engineering or applied physics. To remark simply that the human body is more complex than electrical circuits is to miss the point. What matters is that they represent different kinds of complexity. The international telephone system (taken as a whole) probably has about as many elementary "parts" as the human body has cells. Viewed in some ways (designing, manufacturing, warehousing, assembling), this total system is of staggering complexity. But from the viewpoint we have been developing, the telephone system can be regarded as a relatively simple one. All the electrical processes involved in the system are explicit and known; all are predictable from Maxwell's equations and quantum mechanics. Similarly, all the mechanical operations involved are Newtonian and can be accounted for by a few well-known laws. The construction and maintenance of the system can be accounted for by well-understood economic principles. Indeed, it is the existence of these laws with their power and generality, and the explicitness of the individual processes, which makes it possible to construct and operate such enterprises as the telephone system. It also makes them readily explainable. The mechanical, electrical, and economic theories underlying telecommunications are, in a sense, commensurable. The many different interlocking and elementary processes involved relate to one another, not in some vague or mysterious way but specifically and in detail. These circumstances result from the fact that a telephone system is nowhere near as hierarchically organized as a human being. It is to a very large extent an aggregation of like components, not of unlike ones, and as a result it displays very few emergent properties.

The knowledge structure of medicine is completely different. To begin with, there are few general theories. Instead, we have at best some principles or maxims that seem to have a useful generality, for example, the molecular basis of genetics, the notion of biochemical uniformism, and the evidence of evolution. But most of the powerful laws of science are those that exhibit themselves in a horizontal fashion. Maxwell's equations are most useful at particular descriptive levels. Such laws, however, do not explain matters well when we examine the relations among hierarchical levels. Indeed, we would seem to have almost no laws or rules that describe vertical processes, with perhaps the exception of the evolutionary paradigm. At our present level of medical knowledge, we are unable to perceive the nature of the connections among things in biology in the way that engineers perceive such connections among artifacts.

If, upon observing a patient or learning of a patient's complaint, we do not immediately recognize the disorder or find that the symptoms and signs fall into well-defined categories, we nearly always turn to a causal inquiry. When a set of attributes is not recognized as something previously known, we may take the findings singly and begin an inquiry based upon causation. We ask ourselves, "What can cause upper abdominal pain and blisters upon the skin?" There are several ways in which we may hope to answer questions of this kind. One is simply to have in mind one list of diseases that may cause abdominal pain and another list of diseases in which blisters are seen. We then need only search these lists for the diseases which they have in common. All physicians have such lists in mind. The more successful diagnosticians appear to have very extensive lists, along with some idea of the conditional probabilities involved. The weakness of this method is that human memory is limited, and that uncommon conditions are the most easily overlooked. A second method overcomes this weakness to some extent. Instead of using mental lists of disease attributes, which in themselves may have little mnemonic value, we might better ask, "What kinds of abnormal processes can cause abdominal pain of this particular type?" and "What mechanisms can cause blisters?" Instead of considering the abdomen as an abstract object that can take on certain attributes, we regard it as a space containing particular organs that are engaged in specific processes, and that connect with or are related to one another in known ways. And blisters are not just fluid-filled bumps on the skin, but the result of such causes as friction, photosensitivity, or underlying pathologies in the dermal-epidermal interface. Asking such causal (pathophysiological) questions may then serve to prompt our memories.

The usefulness of causal reasoning in diagnosis is limited by the state of medical knowledge and the physician's familiarity with it. Anatomy and physiology are by now reasonably well-integrated bodies of knowledge but, until fairly modern times this knowledge was limited to affairs ranging between levels 0 and —4 (see fig. 5.1); that is, from the patient as a whole to organ parts. Biochemistry, from the turn of the century until fairly recently, has been almost entirely concerned with matters at levels —7 and —9. In many areas we are still a long way from closing this gap. But explanation in medicine is to a considerable extent a vertical affair, and wide gaps in our knowledge across hierarchies are troublesome. To explain a beating heart requires that we establish connections between levels ranging from —2 to —9.

With the availability of fresh knowledge, improved techniques, and interdisciplinary approaches such as chemical pathology, molecular pharmacology, and neurochemistry, rapid progress is being made in the understanding of some of these interlevel connections. As these connections become better understood, causal reasoning will become an even more powerful diagnostic tool. Scientific medicine is adopting this diagnostic method more and more. And the more this method is used, the greater the importance of individual-case data will become, and the less useful (or needed) the ontologic concept of disease will be. But before this can become the single and exclusive method of diagnosis, we will first need a much more complete explanation of man.

6.5 Other Inference Processes in Diagnosis

We have referred to disease attributes in terms of necessity, sufficiency, and contingency because these terms play specific roles in our information model. Another language has come into increasing use in speaking of disease attributes, and the relations between this language and the language we have been using can be usefully compared. In recent years, a number of writers have drawn the attention of clinicians to a statistical view of laboratory testing, the significance of which has only recently begun to be appreciated. In a number of common situations, our instincts, or hunches, regarding quantitative matters, particularly probabilistic ones, prove to be seriously in error. Such errors resulting from the intuitive process occur more frequently in medicine than we may suppose.

R. S. Galen and S. R. Gambino, in a recent book, stress the importance of one kind of such intuitive error, and use as an example the interpretation of laboratory test results [5]. Three simple concepts are required for this analysis:

1. The *sensitivity* of a particular test, which is defined as the probability that a patient *having* a given disease (D) will produce a positive test result (R); that is, sensitivity $S_e = p(R \mid D)$.

2. The *specificity* of a particular test, which is defined as the probability that a patient *not having* a given disease ($\sim D$) will produce a negative test result ($\sim R$); thus specificity $S_p = p(\sim R \mid \sim D)$.

3. The *prevalence* of the disease (D), which is the fraction (or percentage) of patients *in the population under study* who have the disease (D).

Sensitivity is concerned with the danger of missing a particular disease, or of producing false negative results (type 1 errors). A test with a sensitivity of 100 percent would produce no false negative results; it would never miss detecting disease that is present. Specificity is concerned with the risk of inferring disease where it does not exist; of producing false positive results (type 2 errors). A test with a specificity of 100 percent would yield negative results in all patients who do not have the disease.

For practical purposes, no present laboratory tests are 100 percent sensitive *and* 100 percent specific, although either goal alone can be approached arbitrarily close. It turns out that efforts to increase sensitivity generally have the result of decreasing specificity, and vice versa. The simplest way of thinking about this is to consider what happens if we simply redefine what is meant by "normal." If the upper limit of normal for serum uric acid is taken as 6 mg/dl, the observed sensitivity of the test as an indicator for gout might be about 95 percent. If we were then to redefine "normal" arbitrarily to be less than 5 mg/dl, the sensitivity would increase to perhaps 99 percent. The test would now miss fewer patients who actually had gout. But in so doing it would obviously produce a larger proportion of false positives, so that the greater sensitivity would have been attained at the cost of a reduced specificity.

Why is this important to the clinician? It is important because our intuition in dealing simultaneously with the three factors of sensitivity, specificity, and prevalence is, in practice, found to be unreliable. We can see this by means of the following example, which is taken from S. G. Pauker [92]. Readers who may not have seen this or a similar example before are urged to commit themselves to one of the answers before going on.

Let us take the case of a 35-year-old woman who has been given a new test for breast cancer. It is known that the test has a sensitivity of 95 percent, and a specificity of 90 percent. The prevalence of breast cancer among 35-year-old women will be assumed to be 1 per 1,000. The patient's test result is positive; what is the likelihood that she has breast cancer? (a) Less than 1 percent, (b) about 10 percent, (c) about 40 percent, (d) about 60 percent, (e) about 90 percent, (f) greater than 99 percent. (The answer and a method of analysis is provided in the notes.[8])

Although Galen and Gambino have emphasized the application of this method of analysis to laboratory test results, they do not overlook the generalization that can be made from these concepts. All disease attributes are subject to each of these considerations, and this becomes even more obvious with higher-level attributes. Chest pain is a common symptom of myocardial infarction, but it does not have a test sensitivity of 100 percent; we might assign it a test sensitivity of about 98 percent. However, we would regard it as having a rather low test specificity. It is difficult to estimate a number, but for moderately severe chest pain, which is otherwise not further described, its specificity for myocardial infarction might be somewhere between 10 percent and 20 percent. Pallor or hypotension are also common with this disease, particularly in severe instances, but we would probably not assign a test sensitivity of more than 50 percent, and, for test specificity, much less.

The same analysis is applicable to attributes of this type as to laboratory test results.

Given the facts of the breast cancer case just stated, most physicians (who had not previously thought about the matter) would tend to grossly overestimate the predictive value of the hypothetical test. The reason for this is that they would not have given due weight to the effect of disease prevalence. When this problem is correctly analyzed—which can be done by simple enumeration— the source of the difficulty is readily seen. Once this point is grasped, however, the effect of prevalence must continue to be kept in mind when we examine particular test applications. Galen and Gambino provide a provocative example [5]. Suppose a laboratory test for rheumatoid arthritis has been developed by an investigator who, by using a group of 100 confirmed arthritic patients and a control group of 100 presumed nonarthritic subjects, has determined that the test has a sensitivity of 99 percent and a specificity of 99 percent. The rheumatologists on a hospital staff request the laboratory to make the test available and, after a trial period, they are delighted with the results. Nearly all their patients with rheumatoid arthritis give positive test results, and the false positive test results are rare. In view of this success, it is next proposed that the test be used as a screening procedure for all patients admitted to the hospital. When it is evaluated for this purpose, the false positive rate is found to jump to some 30 percent, and includes patients having a variety of disorders but not one patient with rheumatoid arthritis. This unsatisfactory performance arises because of the low prevalence of rheumatoid arthritis among all patients admitted to the hospital (perhaps 1 percent, compared with the 50 percent prevalence in the population originally investigated, and to a comparable fraction in rheumatologists' own practices). The predictive value of the test,[9] which was 99 percent for the rheumatologists' patients, has now dropped to 50 percent when used as a screening test for all admissions. Half of the positive tests are now false positives. The point of the example is that a test that performs exceedingly well with one specific group of patients having a high prevalence of the disease may be useless for another population in which the disease has a much lower prevalence.

How do the concepts of sensitivity and specificity (as applied to disease attributes) relate to our concepts of necessity, sufficiency, and contingency? First let us consider again the matter of pathognomonic attributes. If we find some patient to have Koplik spots, we would be justified in making the diagnoses of measles (i.e., the sensitivity of this may be reasonably high, although less than 100 percent), because although this attribute *may* be found in this disease it is not found in any others (a selectivity of 100 percent). Since false positives do not occur, the finding has a predictive value (see preceding footnote) of unity. Such findings are sufficient for the diagnosis, but not all patients having this disease need display these findings. The Koplik spots may have vanished by the time the patient with measles is examined, so that the sensitivity of this attribute for measles may be considerably less than 100 percent. Pathognomonic attributes that lie *at high hierarchical levels* tend to have this property.

This particular disease also has necessary attributes; we would not make the diagnosis of measles unless the patient had fever and a macular eruption. Since afebrile cases of measles would be extremely rare, the sensitivity of "fever" for measles would be near 99 percent. Its selectivity for this disease, however, would be very low given the large number of febrile diseases. The sensitivity of an attribute for a given disease, as with necessity, thus requires knowledge of only the disease in question. When the membership criteria for a single class is known, we can tell whether an object belongs to that class or not. Specificity, however, like sufficiency, requires that we have global knowledge, that we have before us the membership criteria for *all* classes in the scheme.

It seems to be for this reason that physicians seem more willing to make estimates of probabilities as $P(A_i \mid D)$ rather than as $P(D \mid A_i)$. A physician's clinical experience is a sequential thing and he will have seen many instances of a common disease (e.g., pneumococcal pneumonia) before he sees a single case of a rare disease (e.g., schistosomiasis, in the U.S.). He is therefore able to use this experience to make some estimate of the probability of a patient having pleuritic pain, given that the patient has pneumococcal pneumonia. He will feel less confident if asked to guess the probability of a patient having schistosomiasis, given that he has diarrhea. Making the latter estimate requires a knowledge of all diseases associated with diarrhea, including knowledge of their distribution and frequency. Nevertheless, physicians are able to diagnose diseases that they have never seen before by resorting to a variety of information sources, and by using what is called "clinical judgment." Just how, then, does judgment work?

7

The Clinical Process

7.1 The Context of Clinical Judgment

Whenever the topic of medical judgment is discussed by physicians and computer scientists, some of the former will be apt to point out that medicine is as much an art as it is a science, and that rules cannot replace intuition and instinct. The computer scientists might then reply that, unless medicine is pure magic, clinical judgment[1] must operate by somehow drawing inferences from patient data and prior knowledge. They will quite correctly point out that certain types of knowledge can be represented in a computer system and that, whether it is operating as a logic engine or as a calculating machine, the computer is more accurate and frequently more rapid than human beings. The debate commonly halts at this point, which is unfortunate because it is precisely at this point that several important issues should be aired.

When these same physicians are again with their medical students, they will likely be found describing the rules for doing this or that and insisting that medicine is a science and not an art. The computer scientist back in his office may resume the task of attempting to represent in his program the difference in meanings of the words *up* and *down,* so that his program will "understand" the sentence "The baby threw up on the down comforter." Serious and interesting issues underlie this debate. Many physicians are in a quandary because they do not quite know what to expect from computers. Perhaps more important, a perceived threat by the computer may have caused some physicians to underestimate the relative worth of their own various skills.

Analysis of the notion of clinical judgment, and of the relationship of computers to judgment in general, involves issues at a number of different levels. We have already examined the differences between low- and high-level objects with respect to the fuzziness and ambiguity involved in their descriptions. There are still other issues: the unanswered questions of how much of judgment is computable, and of whether thought itself is governed by rules. These issues have been analyzed in recent years in terms of "what the computer cannot do" [30], and "what the computer should not do" [135]. Still other writers have found the whole matter simply depressing [67]. To restrict the scope of our discussion in this section, let us consider only the beginning activities of the medical-care process: those occurring from the time of the first patient-physician encounter to the determination of a tentative or working diagnosis.

When a new patient steps into the consultation room, the physician's attention must be fully extended. At that moment, the maximum cognitive span is required of the physician. The primary-care physician must be prepared to deal with the possibility of one or more of several thousand diseases or medical "conditions," and with an unimaginably large number of presentations not representing disease. The results of a preliminary conversation, history-taking, physical examination, and perhaps laboratory tests or special examinations will be used to reduce this enormous set of possibilities to a small number of probable states of affairs—the differential diagnosis. To which of these separate acts, then, are we to apply the term *clinical judgment*? To the selection of the next question, to the search for a particular sign, to the ordering of a diagnostic test, or to the final choice among the alternatives? It might seem equally applicable to all.

Let us represent this judgmental process by a funnel or horn (fig. 7.1), with its large diameter at the onset of the process and its small end at the conclusion. The decreasing diameter of the funnel may be taken to represent the shrinking cognitive span required of the physician during this process. At the start, the physician's breadth of comprehension must extend to the totality of the every-day world.[2] That is, he or she must have at least an average acquaintance with the world and how it works, and must be able to exercise common sense. The necessity for this breadth of comprehension is frequently overlooked as an ingredient in medical judgment. However, in dealing with computer programs nothing

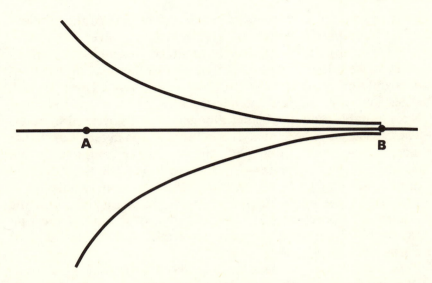

Figure 7.1. Diagram suggesting the breadth of cognitive span required of the physician during a patient encounter. Point A represents the situation when the patient is first seen. Point B, the situation after taking a history and performing a physical examination.

can be taken for granted. And clinical judgment counts for little unless it rests upon a firm base of ordinary human judgment.

Whereas nearly everything is possible at the beginning of a patient visit, the field of possibilities becomes progressively restricted as the visit goes on. As more information is obtained, the possibilities are reduced until only a relatively small number of potential disorders remain as candidates. The cognitive universe, in which further fact finding and inference takes place and in which a decision must finally be made, becomes smaller, more detailed, and more specific. The alternatives not only become fewer but they are sharpened, and relations among them appear. At this point the problem might be said to be well structured.[3]

Although it seems fitting to apply the term *clinical judgment* to the inferential processes occurring between points (A) and (B) (fig. 7.1), these situations appear to be quite different in nature [35]. Some physicians, if pressed about these differences, might reply that the reasoning processes involved near point (B) are the ones most demanding of their abilities; that in this portion of the over-all process their unique skills and detailed knowledge are most called upon, and that here computers would be the least useful. I will argue that the contrary seems actually to be the case.

Let us begin with two examples that are referrable to medical events in the neighborhood of point (B) and which represent problems frequently faced by physicians. One is that of managing the treatment of a patient with acid-base or electrolyte abnormalities. These particular problems lie in an area of medicine in which the causal mechanisms are fairly well understood and the clinical management of a patient has, in part, been reduced to the solution of certain problems in physical biochemistry. The necessary tasks include the taking of a history, the observation of some clinical signs, the determination of particular laboratory data, the substitution of these values into appropriate formulas, and the solution of these formulas. The patient may well have other problems or complaints that are not described by these formulas, and the physician must also deal with them. But a physician who is serious about correcting the acid-base or electrolyte disturbance would do well to use the formulas (at least as a guide to diagnosis and management) since these best capture the current medical understanding of these problems.

In order to facilitate the proper use of these formulas and rules, Howard Bleich has developed computer programs that request and accept certain laboratory and clinical data, solve the problems (with the use of the formulas), and then provide the physician with appropriate advice [11, 12]. Bleich's programs go beyond the arithmetic itself; they may request additional data, suggest a differential diagnosis, make therapeutic suggestions, and explain the basis for the recommendations. It may be asked whether such computer programs perform as well as the physician. Since both the program and the physician in this example employ the same formulas (if they do not always approach the problem identically), perhaps we could phrase the question differently, and ask, "Do physicians solve these formulas (follow these rules) as well as the computer?" Since neither mathematicians nor engineers claim to be able to calculate more reliably than computers, it would seem strange to find physicians who could do so.

Another common clinical problem is that of choosing the proper dose of a drug, particularly with certain relatively toxic ones. Kinetic models of drug distribution (represented as sets of equations) have been developed and incorporated into programs which, when provided with appropriate input data, such as patient weight, renal function, and the amount and timing of the previous drug doses, will then calculate the dose necessary to achieve a desired plasma level [61]. Such a program has been refined through the use of additional techniques, including feedback, in order to deal with idiosyncrasies among patients [49]. When such systems are evaluated, their performance usually appears to be better than the unaided physician's judgment. This should come as no surprise if one grants that, despite limitations which we shall discuss later, computers do *calculate* extremely well. Programs of this type have become known as "expert" or "consultant" systems, although they differ in fundamental ways from other programs employing different techniques, which provide clinical advice in dealing with acute renal failure [93] and antimicrobial therapy [115].

The above examples are concerned with processes that are deterministic in the sense that their behavior can be predicted by known chemical or physical laws. If a relevant law is known and if it can be represented by a suitable formula, a computation seems generally to yield a more accurate prediction than estimation or intuition. But there are nondeterministic (stochastic) processes that on average can be predicted by formulas, whence insurance companies and gambling casinos are profitable.

In 1954, Paul E. Meehl, a clinical psychologist, reviewed a number of different studies in which the performance of a clinician (usually a psychologist) was compared with that of some statistical procedure. These studies were concerned with a variety of tasks, including psychological diagnosis, predicting the performance of entering college freshmen or of student aviators, and the prediction of recidivism among parolees. In each instance, certain test data or historical data were available, and a statistical procedure (frequently as simple as a linear regression procedure) was then applied after it had been empirically fitted to previous information on the particular task. The overall result of Meehl's review was that in each of the twenty-four (later increased to thirty-five) comparison studies the statistical, or as Meehl termed it, the "actuarial" method, performed as well as, or better than, the human predictors [80, 81]. The results of Meehl's studies proved disconcerting to many clinicians and apparently puzzled Meehl himself. We seem instinctively to have a high regard for careful judgment. How could a mindless formula compete with it? As Elstein [35] has commented, these findings appear puzzling, contrary to our intuition, and controversial. Meehl's actuarial methods set standards of performance that could be approached or equaled, but not generally surpassed, by groups of human predictors. Once an optimum prediction formula has been found, using it to find a correct answer seems to be the best method to use. There is no level of performance in calculating that is superior to achieving correctness.

More recently, medical diagnostic algorithms based upon a number of techniques (statistical methods, including pattern matching and clustering procedures, decision rules, and production rules) have been incorporated into computer programs. These have been designed to use observational data and to select the proper alternative from a fixed (and usually small) set of choices. Such diagnostic programs have been used for congenital heart disease [132], thyroid disease [27], and acute abdominal pain [28]. A program of the last type, developed by F. T. DeDombal, has been evaluated in the emergency rooms of several hospitals in Europe. It has been claimed to perform better than house staff physicians and slightly better than consultants when the same clinical information is made available to both the program and a clinician. Performances such as these have been viewed by many physicians either with skepticism or as a prospective threat. Such results again raise questions of the nature and role of clinical judgment.

In considering this matter it is essential to appreciate that these prediction or decision programs (like those cited by Meehl) deal with activities located near point (B)[4] of figure 7.1. All of these computer programs operate in small and well-structured task domains, which were initially organized (formalized) by a human judge functioning earlier at point (A). This feature is nearly always overlooked in discussions of computer diagnosis. Questions such as "Do we run the acute abdominal pain program, or the chest pain program?" or even "Shall we run a diagnostic program?" must first be decided by human beings. A great deal of human information processing must take place before the job can be turned over to a computer. When Michael Scriven writes (of Meehl's results) "The ultimate ignominy is surely to discover that the vast experience and formal training of the clinician results in judgments no better than the simplest possible formula...," he repeats this error [111]. By failing to recognize where the judgmental process begins, he confuses a portion of a process (the final choice among well-defined alternatives) with an entire process.

But let us go back and examine the informational state of affairs at point (A). How many facts are there here? Asking this question is equivalent to asking how many facts would have to be listed if one were to attempt a complete description of the world. Researchers in artificial intelligence, cognitive psychologists, and philosophers have considered this matter in much more detail than can be recounted here. Among the optimists, workers in artificial intelligence such as Marvin Minsky have estimated that something like a million "facts" would be needed to achieve "great intelligence" in an artificial intelligence system[5] [26]. Earlier, Russell and Wittgenstein (in his *Tractatus*), proposed that the world might be susceptible to description in terms of "atomic statements," propositions so primitive that they would require no further explanation. This hope (for logical atomism) was subsequently abandoned by most philosophers, including Wittgenstein, and it now seems generally agreed that there is no way of avoiding an infinite regress if one attempts to describe the world in this way. In other words, *any* fact statement or proposition will raise further questions that require still further explanations, which lead to still more questions, ad infinitum. The everyday world, it appears, not only cannot be described by a small number of *primitive* statements (there being no such things) but neither can be described by a finite number of any kind of statement.

As we have already seen, the number of things that can be truthfully said about any object in the world is unimaginably large, and the only way in which we can speak usefully of things is to confine ourselves to matters that count (i.e., are relevant). By relevant, I mean connected to the topic or purpose with which we are engaged at a given moment. It is only through this selection of relevant attributes that we succeed in communicating at all. At point (A), almost all the things that could be attributed to a patient would be irrelevant to the problem of finding out what is wrong. It is the physician's task to select from this unimaginably large number of indifferent and neutral facts the ones that happen to be relevant. This situation is quite unlike the one at point (B) where this selection process is largely completed, expert knowledge alone may suffice, and where a calculation may do the trick. Once point (B) is reached in the process of clinical judgment, the irrelevant facts have been filtered out, and the medical problem has become relatively well structured. But initially the funnel of required comprehension is wide open, interfacing with the world in all its complexity.

How does the physician deal with this complexity, and how successful are computer programs at this task? Many distinguished physicians have taught that history-taking is the most critical step in the entire diagnostic process, and that performance in this is what separates the exceptional physician from the less able. From the viewpoint of information theory, this idea seems quite plausible. Consider the manner in which we go about measuring the difference between the diagnostic worth of a fact that is volunteered by a patient and a fact that is elicited in response to a question. In CMIT, as we have seen, 3,262 diseases and "medical conditions" are listed, with each defined in terms of clinical and laboratory attributes. In our studies of this compilation, the term *nosebleed* (or its synonyms) was found to occur in the description of 27 different diseases. If a new patient voluntarily complained of "nosebleed," our attention would be drawn to these 27 diseases, and not to the 3,235 of which "nosebleed" is not considered to be a characteristic. If, however, we were routinely to ask every patient we saw whether or not he or she had "nosebleed," the great majority of replies would be negative, and this information would allow us to reject (or set aside) only 27 diseases instead of 3,235. The "diagnostic" or "selection" power of a positive response, in this example, is thus more than a hundredfold greater than a negative one. And when patients volunteer facts, these facts are almost always stated in an affirmative sense. Patients do not complain of symptoms that they do *not* have. The amount of information obtained from a random inquiry about symptoms (and obtaining for the most part negative responses) will therefore be very small. If, in contrast, the patient is encouraged to volunteer affirmative (positive) symptoms, the information value is clearly much greater. Every practitioner knows and practices this instinctively, although it is not widely appreciated that this method rests upon a firm theoretical basis. By beginning in this way (with the "chief complaint") the physician, equipped with both common sense and medical knowledge, is provided with a means for exploiting relevance. This is the physician's method for dealing with the unimaginably complex. How well would computer programs do here?

Perhaps the only computer programs relevant to this particular point are those designed to take the patient's medical history [119].

When introduced some years ago, these programs appeared to offer great promise, but since then interest in them has waned. R. B. Friedman and D. H. Gustafson have commented,

> A graphic example [of the failure to report the reasons for unsuccessful system performance] can be found in the area of computer applications to the acquisition of Medical History Data. Numerous groups across the country have worked and published in this area, often duplicating previous efforts. However, although the great majority of these efforts have since been abandoned we could find no publications detailing the reasons for these failures. (*Comput. Biomed. Res.* [1977] 8:199-204)

Yet the cause for this failure does not seem too difficult to locate. In order to ask *relevant* questions of a patient, the physician uses his or her sense of the situation and general medical knowledge. But for a fact to be relevant, it must have some demonstrable bearing upon something, and, by deciding that a fact is relevant, a physician has already started the process of diagnosis. We cannot collect relevant data without having a theory or diagnosis in mind, despite suggestions that data collection and diagnosis can be carried out as separate enterprises. G. Anthony Gorry has pointed out the limitations of programs based on decision analysis alone, and has alluded to the role of commonsense knowledge [48] (see also [124]).

For the most significant portions of the medical history, even current computer programs having substantial breadth (although they may follow a systematic course) can at best ask rote questions and will, for the most part, obtain low-worth, negative responses. Moreover, even when positive responses are obtained with these systems, clinicians have complained that they require further investigation, and that the information so obtained frequently turns out to be unimportant [51, 73, 76]. This type of performance is to be expected when the issue of relevance has been ignored. Several studies have confirmed that these automated systems for obtaining medical histories usually obtain "valid" information. But irrelevancy, not invalidity, is the source of the problem, and determining what is relevant in a clinical situation requires common sense and general medical knowledge.

As far as the performance of judgmental (as opposed to computational) processes is concerned, the everyday problems around point (A) appear to be the ones with which computer programs are least useful. Indeed, it is doubtful that they have ever performed there. To put it differently, for a computer program to perform successfully in this region it would be necessary for the programmer to have developed a means of representing the universe of possibilities at this point. And at point (A) this would entail a description of the world comparable in extent to human commonsense knowledge. Artificial intelligence researchers who work with programs that attempt to "understand" natural language [140], or to provide expert advice [19, 116], have devised ingenious and impressive systems. These appear to perform reasonably well, however, only when operating in so-called microworlds; that is, within extremely small task domains that are near point (B) and have been carefully structured and circumscribed. Only in this way can the builder hope to supply the necessary a priori knowledge. Some of these point (B) systems have proven very useful [19], and others have shown promise [84, 115].[6] The expectation, however, that the real world at point (A) can be reconstructed from a large set of these microworlds has not received any support, and would seem on epistemological grounds to be in serious doubt [16, 30].[7]

There appear to be two principal approaches open for the development of computer programs that could be said to "behave intelligently." By behave intelligently I mean be able to operate successfully nearer to point (A) than to point (B), and to deal with a variety of ordinary life situations.[8] The first of these requires a means to represent commonsense knowledge in a computer program so that it could be applied to raw situations. So far, progress in achieving this goal has been scant and the problem may, as has been suggested, be intractable. An alternative to storing such a priori knowledge would be to devise a program that would be, in a realistic sense, capable of "learning." But the kind of learning needed includes the generalization of what has been learned. This has not been accomplished after some thirty years of effort [86].

There may be a third approach, which would render the entire issue moot. This would be the discovery of yet unknown technologies—of hardware, architecture, and software so radically different from anything presently known that a system using them could in some sense be said to "live." By living in the world (surviving, competing, succeeding, failing, and so on) such a device might begin to acquire knowledge on its own. Whether the development of such a system is possible, and what we would call it if it were invented, will not be considered here.

The essential issue is to distinguish between the nature of the situations existing at point (A), where the totality of the world must be confronted, and those at point (B), where the task domain has already been structured through previous human effort, an abstraction is available, and little commonsense knowledge may be required. My reason for emphasizing this difference is that the physician, equipped with medical knowledge through training and experience, and with commonsense knowledge from having lived in the world, can readily deal with the first situation. Physicians can obviously perform well at point (B), too, although there are a growing number of specific (and computable) processes being programmed in this region that will enable a computer to outperform physicians at this point. This trend is certain to continue.

It would be unfortunate, therefore, if physicians were to mistakenly regard their professional cognitive skills as lying in just those steps of the diagnostic process which are, or may become, computational in nature, and thereby minimizing their indispensable role in dealing with situations generally. This seems a process far beyond the present or foreseeable reach of the computer. It seems to be only in highly structured and formalized situations that we are presented with choices between human beings and machines; our more interesting problems involve the selection of appropriate roles for human beings *and* machines. And in this selection it would not seem presumptuous to suggest that each be used for the things which they perform best, particularly since these tasks appear to be quite different.

7.2 Performance and Purpose

The earliest applications of electronic digital computers were in the performance of arithmetic tasks. The first among these modern machines (ca. 1940-1950), were constructed by teams of mathematicians and engineers having difficult computing jobs at hand. Typically, these jobs involved solving complex equations in engineering, ballistics, hydrodynamics, or nuclear physics. Although the applicability of such machines to the solutions of logic problems, and to information processing tasks more generally, had been long foreseen, the early machines were almost exclusively put to work in numerical computing. These vacuum tube (before that, relay or punched-tape) machines, programmed with difficulty and operating unreliably ("down time" exceeded "running time" for several years), were suitable primarily for research work. Yet it had been clear from the beginning that with greater reliability they would find application in many other fields. In the decade 1950 to 1960, with the development of markedly improved primary and secondary storage devices, and specialized peripheral devices (e.g., magnetic tape readers, magnetic discs, printers, and methods for reading magnetically recorded account numbers on checks), they found their use first in banking and insurance, and shortly thereafter in commerce more generally. During this same period, the development of programming languages made feasible the construction of large-scale custom computing systems, and gave birth to the modern software industry.

This transition in application from scientific computing, where the programmer, operator, and ultimate user of the machine were frequently the same person, to commercial applications (where the designers, developers, managers, and users included a number of different kinds of people) gave rise to unanticipated difficulties. It seems to have been expected that the computerization of many common and routine processes, which were subject to careful definition (bookkeeping, accounting, billing, etc.), could be accomplished by a straightforward extension of the techniques that had proven satisfactory in scientific computing. This expectation was not fulfilled. Although commercial processes are to a large extent numerical ones, they involve much more than that. Commerce requires a knowledge of more than arithmetic. Customers may not pay their bills on time, or they may erroneously pay them twice. Individual behavior and the behavior of the marketplace are not governed by known laws, and neither are completely predictable. Certain features of the everyday world are interwoven with these processes, and some absurd results were produced by early computer systems because their designers had overlooked this fact. Many of the anecdotes concerning the stupidity of computers had their origin in this period when customers had their electrical service improperly turned off for alleged lack of payment, were repeatedly billed for something they'd already paid for, or received multiple copies of the same magazine. The necessity for dealing with exceptions began to be recognized by system designers, and the many corrections and adjustments that humans have always contributed to these processes became more fully appreciated when computers took over these processes. As C. West Churchman put it, "it is no easy matter to make a computer behave as a clerk would do" [23]. The further extension in the use of computers from commerce to such recent applications as decision making and "question answering" systems represents a third phase in the evolution of computers, and these new applications have raised still different problems. It will be noted that something quite systematic has occurred during these three stages. The mathematical problems involved in scientific computation are complete abstractions to begin with. A program competent to deal with abstractions requires only what are known as a set of "effective procedures" and the data. There is no need for any general knowledge of the world; indeed, as we have already seen, there is no way for mathematics to deal with such knowledge. In contrast, many commercial applications involve *incomplete* abstractions of the world. Although most of what these programs accomplish can be done by working with complete abstractions alone, some world knowledge and a means for using it becomes necessary in order to deal with exceptions. It would not do for a health insurance company to pay benefits for hysterectomies in successive years on behalf of the same patient, or to pay pregnancy benefits to a single male subscriber. Although avoiding such results as these is simple, it is necessary that relevant knowledge about the world be provided to the system, because these empirical facts are not deducible from the axioms of mathematics or logic. This is easier said than done, since what counts as relevant depends upon the particularity of situations, and considerable foresight on the part of system designers is required. At the third stage, when something approximating "intelligent behavior" is attempted, the issues of relevance and abstraction become particularly difficult.

An important question in medicine is how we can distinguish between the processes that seem appropriate for machines and those that are more suitable for human performance. In the previous section I proposed a metaphor to represent the changing cognitive span required of a physician upon being consulted by a new patient. My purpose was to emphasize the differences between raw situations in the world (point A) and the well-structured problems which humans are able to abstract from such situations, and which may then be suitable for computation (point B). Although the context employed was that of medical diagnosis, the process itself is a more general one. After all, no matter what we may be doing at a given moment, we are always at point (A) with respect to an infinitude of other and different activities we could elect to undertake. The directions along which we depart point (A) will depend upon our intentions, goals, or plans.

It would seem that computers are likely to be of least help to us at point (A), in the early phases of activities during which we recognize problems, assemble facts, set goals and, in general, analyze situations. In this activity we might appear to be choosing one thing over another, and it is tempting to regard some of it as decision making. Yet we never start with decisions, unless someone has first formalized a problem for us. Decision making occurs at point (B).

The initial groping among things and sorting out of affairs, which goes on at point (A), are characteristic activities of living organisms, and are especially characteristic of humans. People seem to be most comfortable when these groping and sorting out activities are entrusted to humans. With the well-structured problems at point (B), however, we find many opportunities for taking advantage of the two most powerful properties of a computer: its speed of processing and its capacity for storing extremely large quantities of data. If our problems can be formalized, and if an effective procedure is available, the solution may then be obtained as a computation. Many of the "expert" or diagnostic programs cited in the previous section, and all of the "arithmetic" types of medical programs (computerized tomography, physiological monitoring and data reduction, radiotherapy planning) are performed as computations of this kind. Many of these point (B) computations are carried out automatically, with human involvement being limited to supplying the data, monitoring the performance of the system, and collecting the solutions.

7.3 The Formalization of Ordinary Situations

We have used the term *artificial intelligence* at several points without further explanation, and it is time now to consider what it is that seems to be meant by this term. It is sometimes said that artificial intelligence (AI) means the accomplishment by a computer program of purposes that would otherwise require human intellectual activity. But this would not seem to reflect what other AI workers really intend. They would not consider a computer program that merely does arithmetic as being AI, although it meets the above requirement. Nor would they so regard a program for finding a new prime number, even though this activity almost surpasses human capabilities. However, a program that plays checkers or chess, or one that turns on a green light when the message "turn on the green light" is typed in, would be considered as AI. It is not easy to state in advance what would count as an AI project.

Workers in the field of AI at the present time have a considerable diversity of motivations and techniques. The goals they address are similarly diverse. Some deal with problems of long-standing interest, such as general machine translation or language understanding, and others have practical, short-term ends. Among the latter are projects concerned with the development of programs for assisting with everyday problems. These include medical diagnosis, natural language processing, image or picture processing, and the construction of automatic machinery or robots. Since many of these activities can be carried out to some degree by ordinary algorithmic programs, the features that best characterize AI projects are (1) those that make use of heuristic programs (sets of rules, the use of which is hoped to provide an acceptable performance, though not promising to yield a single "correct" answer), (2) attempts to use prestored knowledge, in order to make inferences about a particular problem domain, and (3) programs that can "learn" and thus improve their performance when the same or similar task is repeated. One particularly successful program of this type, DENDRAL, is used by chemists to identify unknown molecular structures from the data obtained with mass spectroscopy and nuclear magnetic resonance spectroscopy. The designers of these systems have not, for the most part, made the explicit claim that their programs simulate the processes that humans employ in carrying out these activities, nor have they insisted that the study of their programs need shed light upon the nature of the corresponding human processes. This subdivision of AI is increasingly being referred to as "knowledge engineering."

Other researchers prominent in the development of the field have had rather different goals. Some have espoused "information processing" theories of the human mind: the hypothesis that human mental processes can be formalized and simulated with computer programs. Some holding this view have claimed that a major portion of future psychology research will involve the study of computer programs. Still others appear to have had as their objective the imitation of human cognitive activities. It is not clear how much of this latter activity is to be seriously taken as having an explanatory value in understanding nature and, therefore, to be construed as a scientific undertaking rather than as a game. On balance, it seems that some of the present activities in the field of AI are beginning to become a part of conventional science, whereas others are not. In a field as new and full of ferment as AI, it is not surprising to find such an assortment of goals and expectations.[9]

One particular type of AI activity has occasioned criticism. Without having the aim of seeking to understand some aspect of human behavior, some researchers have attempted to imitate it more in appearance than in performance. An early example of such a program was Joseph Weizenbaum's ELIZA, an interactive program that creates the illusion that the user is conversing with a psychiatrist. It was Weizenbaum's surprise at discovering that people appeared so willing to succumb to this illusion that prompted him to write his well-known criticism of AI [135]. Some of the illusionists appear to justify their work on the grounds that the man-computer interaction may be facilitated by fostering the impression that there is a human being participating in the process. Still other researchers seem more motivated by the prospect of successfully tricking people, and to this extent they are playing games. McCorduck suggests that these and other motives may be closely interwoven [77].

One of the features necessary in most AI programs is some representation of world knowledge. If AI programs are to deal with real situations, one school believes it is necessary initially to delimit sufficiently the small domain or piece of the world in which the program is intended to function. Several different approaches have been tried. One has been to attempt to isolate a small piece of the everyday world that contains some particular features of interest, and which is thought to be of a manageable size. Schank, for example, in one of his earlier projects made the assumption that the activities which occur in a limited and presumably stereotyped arena (he used the example of a restaurant) might be represented in a program by means of "scripts," which would describe the typical activities occurring in such a domain [108]. The central idea was that most of the activities occurring in a restaurant are repetitious and hence formalizable. For example, a customer enters, is seated, is handed a menu, makes a selection, and so on. The nonstereotypical happenings that might arise would be handled as exceptions. His program would then be expected to reach certain conclusions not explicitly given, but deducible from the stated circumstances. For example, if a customer ordered a steak, and later paid for it, the program would infer that he had eaten it. The difficulty with this kind of approach in practice seems to be that since the a priori knowledge provided is necessarily incomplete, the exceptions quickly come to dominate matters. This is not surprising if we reflect upon the nature of everyday affairs. Since a customer can do many of the things in a restaurant that he can do elsewhere, and the things he cannot do there (e.g., hang-gliding) he can speak of, plan for, or conspire about, the program must, in effect, be prepared for everything. Failing this, its performance will appear unrealistic and gamelike. But this is just what a program cannot do, and why the microworld was constructed in the first place. This procedure of attempting to construct a microworld either fails to sever the connections between the model and the world, or behaves in an artificial and unrealistic manner. We have already noted that there is no systematic way of counting or enumerating facts about the world. Hence there is no way for a designer to know whether or not he has left some facts out, or to determine how many more facts need be listed. There is no such thing as "the next fact." There are as many "facts" involved in the restaurant microworld as there are in the world itself, and the attempted demarcation fails. This approach, which attempts to decompose the world into sets of distinct microworlds, is an attempt at the analytic demarcation of human experience. The experiences, with logical atomism would suggest this to be a futile direction in which to proceed.

An alternative approach is to take single facts or propositions, one at a time, and by using sufficient numbers of them attempt to create a coherent and closed domain. This is the method employed in mathematics, and it is used in the construction of all game-playing programs. Here there are no connections between these newly created programs and the world because none is introduced.

The resulting artificial domain is therefore subject only to rules of the creator's choice. Unlike the former procedure, this one yields manageable descriptions, though the domain itself may be an impoverished one with little resemblance to the real world. The distinction between these approaches is useful because those AI projects, which had had practical objectives and have proven most useful, would seem to be of the second type. Whether this will continue to be the case depends on the outcome of the many current attempts to describe formally significant portions of the everyday world, and to deal with the problem of representing commonsense knowledge. There is considerable controversy as to whether such attempts are well founded, or even possible in principle [16, 30]. Nevertheless, in dealing with certain highly structured or formalizable situations (which are most apt to be found at low hierarchical levels), there seems little doubt that useful tools can be constructed in this general manner.

7.4 Tasks for People and Tasks for Machines

In the process that extends from the physician's initial involvement in a situation to the recognition of a problem, its subsequent formalization and, finally, to its solution, we have focused primarily upon the beginning and the end of the process. At the very beginning (point A), the first task is to make sense of a situation, "to let Mind introduce order into chaos." We do this in medicine by using our experience in dealing with ordinary life-situations, and by drawing upon our common sense and general medical knowledge. These preliminary steps, upon which the success of all else depends, appears to require the cognitive breadth found only in humans. Toward the end of this process, when a particular problem has been isolated and formalized, and a solution is being sought, computational or other informational aids may make important contributions. We have stressed these extremes in an attempt to distinguish between functions that, on the one hand, appear to have an absolute requirement for human cognition, and those on the other, which may be performed not only successfully but in many cases better, by machines.

Much of a physician's effort is spent at neither of these two extremes, but is occupied with activities lying between them. The questions then arise, "How far to the left of point (B) are computer aids likely to be helpful to the physician?" and "What will be their nature?" Since a great deal of a physician's time and effort is expended at present in gathering together medical records, X-ray films, and laboratory data, perhaps we should distinguish between "management support" and "informational support" systems. This is not a sharp division, but let us say that computer systems that perform primarily such housekeeping functions as patient registration, appointment scheduling, the communication of medical orders within a hospital, and the generation of a laboratory technician's work schedules, are management support systems. They are characterized by the fact that they do not require the use of significant amounts of medical knowledge. These systems would operate pretty much in the same way, whether the medical data were based upon eighteenth-century medical knowledge or twentieth-century medical knowledge. This is in no way meant to minimize the importance of these activities to the safe and effective care of patients. The greater part of our present medical information systems are, in fact, of this type. When physicians were asked what they believed would be the most useful application of computers in their own practices or hospitals, it was most frequently these kinds of housekeeping applications (particularly record-keeping systems) that they suggested.[10] This attitude is easy to understand. Most physicians find satisfaction in taking care of patients, and are put off by routine paperwork. If housekeeping functions could be turned over entirely to computers—and substantial numbers of them eventually will be—they would be greatly pleased.

We will not consider these medical management systems in any detail here because they have been reviewed elsewhere [70], and because they largely improve the efficiency of conventional and well-understood procedures. Instead, we will consider a group of medical information systems that are designed to provide support to the physician with respect to their *professional* cognitive activities. In particular, we will consider systems that attempt to provide the kinds of help that a physician might hope to receive in discussing a patient's case with a colleague, a specialist consultant, or a medical librarian. This kind of assistance does not yet rank very high on the average physician's list of things he would like a computer to do for him. This may be partly because these activities are a bit too close to the things a physician is expected to do for himself, and which he enjoys doing. There also seems to be an important misconception involved—a physician may feel he is being replaced to some degree by a computer system rather than perceiving the system as a tool to extend and amplify his skills. This misconception has been encouraged by some computer advocates, who envision computer systems as cognitive replacements for physicians rather than as consultants or decision aids. The important differences between using the computer as a tool and the notion of the computer as an automaton or substitute human will be taken up in chapter 10. The more significant reason for physicians' lack of interest (at least until the present) is that medical computer programs have offered the physician very little. As more useful systems are developed, this attitude can be expected to change, and early evidence of this change can now be perceived.

What then of the interval between points (A) and (B)? What of the processes in which a human and a computer might be cooperatively engaged, a task that would be regarded as one requiring medical knowledge if the human were performing it alone? Several such programs have been developed, the most interesting of which are termed *interactive*. These programs not only permit the computer to accept initial data but go on to request additional data or instructions, as appropriate, at intermediate stages of a process. This allows the human user to intervene, to influence the course of a process, and to verify its performance. Most of these interactive programs have fairly limited goals, and they all fall far short of using, or involving, the human partner to best advantage. The human's contribution has usually been limited to entering specifically requested data, and the initiative throughout the interaction resides completely in the program. This is the case with the sophisticated MYCIN program, which asks clinical questions of the user. When MYCIN prints out the question, "Did the patient have the infection before entering the hospital?" it is attempting to determine whether the patient's infection is a hospital-acquired one. To answer this question properly, the physician-user of the system will have to deal with a situation in the world. He may have to distinguish among the following: whether the patient acquired the infection at home, during a previous hospitalization at a different hospital, while on a foreign trip, or whether the patient may be a bacteriologist working in an infectious disease laboratory. Even though the program retains the initiative throughout the interaction, and the user is treated as a passive supplier of data, providing the requested data will require both medical knowledge and cognitive processing.

A different situation occurs in the use of the MEDLINE bibliographic retrieval system.[11] Here a user formulates an inquiry by first selecting the subject area of interest. This is done with the use of standardized indexing terms by means of which original articles were indexed. These terms may then be taken in Boolean combinations in order to express a user's needs: "cancer and cats" would select articles that had been indexed under both terms; "cancer and not cats" would select papers indexed under "cancer" unless they had also been indexed under "cats."

A common search term like "cancer," if employed alone, would obviously bring in an enormous number of citations. No one could ever read all the journal articles dealing with cancer. An inquirer interested in this subject would more likely begin with a more restrictive term like "carcinoma," and then perhaps limit it with "breast." But this might still be too broad a specification, so the search would be further restricted to particular years of publication or language of publication, or by means of additional terms like "chemotherapy" or "etiology." When such a request is processed, MEDLINE first reports the number of articles that satisfy the search criteria. If this number is small, the list of citations and, in some cases, abstracts of the papers as well can be printed out upon request. If the number is too great for printing out on-line (at the user's terminal), a sample of them may be printed out to see if they appear to meet the user's need. If the search appears successful, the listings are printed off-line (printed later on a remote printer) and forwarded by mail, or the user might at this point discover that both clinical and animal studies were included and decide to eliminate the latter. In this recursive process the user can modify, redirect, or entirely respecify the search strategy by manipulating search terms while observing the progress of the system. With such a system, the initiative lies wholly with the user, who is guided in the formulation of subsequent searches by the responses obtained to previous ones. In some institutions where this service is provided (e.g., the libraries of medical schools), an experienced librarian is available to assist in the formulation of inquiries, and the effectiveness of the search will depend on the skill and experience of the user.

The degree of automaticity displayed by a computer system is useful in distinguishing between two types of applications (exemplified here by MYCIN and MEDLINE). There are machines that respond with a uniform level of performance to all users capable of successfully operating them. An adding machine behaves in this way. The other type, exemplified by interactive data-base retrieval systems, although responding to all users, offers the promise of improved performance in the hands of a skillful user.

The first type of system—the "vending machine" type—dispenses a uniform product to all users having the minimum skill needed to operate it. Systems of the interactive type are more like ordinary tools. They require a greater skill in order to use them but, by extending or amplifying the skill of users, they permit human creativity, imagination, and personal knowledge to enter into the achievement of the goal. Man-machine combinations of this second kind, which can more fully utilize the human skills of the user (and, in "default," operate solely on the basis of stored a priori knowledge), will have many useful medical applications in the interval between points (A) and (B).

What kinds of specific tools would facilitate the physician's activities during the process of patient workup? It will first be granted that the majority of patients seen in a primary physician's office present medical problems that are either straightforward or minor. Such cases do not send the physician to the medical library or cause him to call in a consultant. Some will not require even the simplest laboratory procedures. Special tools or services will not be called for with all patients, and it would be regarded as unnecessary and intrusive if they were to be brought in. But in each day's list of patients there may be a few who raise significant questions in the physician's mind. Some of these may be patients not responding appropriately to prescribed medications; patients, for example, with poorly controlled hypertension or diabetes. Each physician will have his own personal strategy for dealing with these patients, perhaps by changing drugs, or adjusting doses. But if these attempts fail, the physician may then need further information, perhaps about a new antihypertensive drug or about types of insulin resistance. Or perhaps he may wish to start all over again, and reevaluate the entire case. Access to the current medical literature is an important support service, and one used to varying degrees by all physicians. Unfortunately, a means for conveniently conducting a rapid and focused search of the current literature is not yet widely available. It seems certain, however, that newly emerging secondary storage technology (perhaps video disks), or information sources available via data networks, will make this a reality before long.[12]

During the course of a week's practice, the primary care physician will also see a few patients with problems that may fully extend his diagnostic skills. Some patients will have disorders resistant to straightaway diagnosis (e.g., a fever of unknown origin) and may require hospitalization and more extensive investigation. Other patients' disorders will be diagnosed in the office, but only after a series of laboratory tests and revisits. With these patients, physicians might well benefit from another kind of information support. One of the strong appeals of computer-based diagnostic programs is that they may suggest diagnoses which the physician has overlooked. This is most likely to occur when the disease in question is uncommon or, if it is a common one, when it presents in an unusual way. The purpose of such systems may not be so much to inform the physician of something of which he is totally unaware as to bring to mind something he may not have thought of or with which he may not be completely familiar. Diagnosis is rarely conducted by physicians as a two-stage process of data collection and inference, despite the fact that some diagnostic programs operate that way. The physician, after making only one or two observations, will begin to create hypotheses that can account for them. He will then seek further evidence that will be confirming or disconfirming of these early hypotheses, and with this new information at hand he will modify his list and begin again. This overall process is rich in possibilities for computer assistance because its recursive nature requires the continuing selection and input of data, and a continuing reevaluation of the current decisions. We will consider several such programs in the next chapter.

Another useful role for computers is in guiding the patient workup in certain information-rich situations. The choice of which clinical evidence to obtain next is one that physicians do without great difficulty, though they probably do not always go about it in the most efficient way. Physicians have not been highly motivated until recently to try to improve their methods. The overuse or inappropriate scheduling of routine diagnostic tests ordinarily poses no hazards for the patient, although such tests may be bothersome or uncomfortable. They may, however, significantly increase the costs of medical care. To the extent that inappropriate or poorly scheduled testing may delay diagnosis, it will also delay treatment and, for the hospitalized patient, result in substantial and avoidable costs. In the later stages of the diagnostic workup, there may be many opportunities to find well-structured problems. It has been shown in the case of the anemias, for example, that once anemia is established the determination of the type of anemia can be determined algorithmically in many cases. This can be done by the stepwise selection of appropriate laboratory tests, which are chosen on the basis of all the information available at a particular time [37]. If this process is computable, a program can use the known information most effectively, and minimize the time and cost of arriving at the diagnosis. A physician once aware of the anemia may, of course, hit upon the correct diagnosis immediately by acquiring higher-level attributes: questioning may establish that the patient is a food faddist with an iron deficiency anemia, or careful physical examination may suffice for the diagnosis of pernicious anemia. On the whole, however, studies of physicians' test planning in diagnosing anemias have shown that the test sequences used are frequently less than optimal.

A second general kind of information need involves the acquisition of new knowledge. For this, the main limitation of the literature is that, even if the literature can be accessed efficiently and successfully, the information available typically consists of generalizations about diseases, diagnoses, and treatments. The practicing physician, in contrast, is always faced with a particular patient having specific problems. The need is for information relevant in this special context.

The presentation of diseases, their course and recommended therapies, as described in textbooks and monographs, are necessarily stated as generalizations. It may be difficult to particularize this information to a given sex, age range, race, or occupational group to the stage of the disease in question or to the presence or absence of other common diseases. This is inevitable because such specific information is simply unavailable for each of these permutations, and the abstractions performed in assembling the data have omitted these particulars. Without such abstractions, the amount of information would be so great as to be unmanageable.

Detail of this degree cannot be represented in textbook form. But the management of large volumes of information is a task for which computers are particularly well suited, and here the computer offers particular promise to medicine.

One of the better known of the projects that have dealt with this is the American Rheumatology Association Medical Information System (ARAMIS) of James Fries [41]. This approach records the clinical and laboratory findings for individual patients having a limited number of disorders (rheumatoid arthritis, scleroderma, lupus erythematosus, and dermatomyositis) and store these data in what Fries has called a "time-oriented data base." The clinical status and course of the patients are recorded in terms of ordinary clinical terminology and laboratory values, and their outcomes under various treatments are likewise recorded. When a new patient with one of these diseases has been fully worked up, and the choice of treatment is under consideration, the outcomes of previous patients who *closely resemble* the current patient in relevant respects can be scrutinized under the various treatments used, and a suitable treatment chosen for the new patient. This procedure permits the matching of a new patient, not with an exemplar or a generalization but with actual sets of individual patients whose outcomes are known. This overcomes the weaknesses inherent in working with generalizations, which may match too easily because they contain too few particulars. This project exemplifies a balanced partnership in which the physician's capability to select and describe relevant patient attributes in specific situations is combined with the computer's effectiveness at storing, managing, and searching large volumes of detailed clinical data. This type of system, designed to provide *specific* medical information to a physician, requires a large-scale clinical data base in which carefully standardized patient data have been recorded. As computer hardware costs continue to decline, and as experience is gained with this and similar systems, this approach will become increasingly effective in providing specific medical information.

There is, finally, a third information function of importance. Where does clinical knowledge come from in the first place? How do medical textbooks get written? The necessary source data come ultimately from individual patient records. And the creation and interpretation of these records depends on the organizing principles prevailing in today's state of medical knowledge. So we must also inquire into the processes that might link a knowledge-base system to a clinical data-base system. The opportunity of accomplishing this has not been widely recognized.[13] Practicing physicians, of course, carry out this process all the time, mostly subconsciously. They employ their basic medical knowledge in the care of their patients, and their subsequent experience with these same patients is then used to modify this knowledge. Whether a deeper analysis of this linking process can lead to the development of comprehensive computer-based tools remains to be seen, but there is much current interest in this possibility. The opportunities for the development of useful information tools of the three general types we have discussed would in any case seem to be particularly encouraging. How we can systematically go about identifying these opportunities will be the subject of the remainder of the book.

8

The Creation of
Medical Information

8.1 On Inquiry and the Discovery of Facts

Before taking up the matter of what it is that moves us to make observations and organize inquiries, it should be understood that neither facts nor answers are just lying about out there in the world for us to stumble across. We sometimes behave as though they were. We may talk about "data collection," or "gathering" clinical information as though we were speaking of sweeping leaves or picking up pebbles on the beach. Sometimes, too, we regard problem solving as an early task rather than a late one; as though problems came to us already packaged and labeled. Such things as data, facts, and problems do not, of course, exist until we have first put our minds to work. Polanyi put it this way,

> ... nothing is a problem or discovery in itself; [something] can be a
> problem only if it puzzles and worries somebody, and a discovery
> only if it relieves somebody of the burden of a problem. [97]

Medical data and clinical information come into existence because someone has been "puzzled" or "worried," and then only after certain particular things have been noticed and formalized. In this crucial sense, clinical data and medical information are always created. Their creation begins when we focus our attention upon one feature rather than another, when we pay attention to the distended neck veins and not to the necktie. Medical information processes begin with these theory-laden observations carried out within situations, and if we begin to delve into some single fact too quickly, we may miss its connections with everything else. Creating information is to be distinguished from the mere acts of noting, measuring, or recording something. The creation of a laboratory test result begins when a physician feels he has some reason for ordering a particular test for a patient and does so, not when a technician performs the test, or when the result is written on a laboratory slip. When we order a particular test (or ask a patient a specific question, or look for a physical sign), we do so because we have made a mental commitment that it is *this particular thing* that we wish to know about, and not something else. Such sought for facts are very different from data that may be provided to us when we have not asked for it, such as the results of screening tests. The former are different because they arise in response to an interest in, or need for, *specific* information. When we are told things we have not asked to be told we are faced with a totally different issue —that of deciding relevance.

What moves us to go about this process of clinical inquiry? We might as well ask what it is that moves us to find out anything at all. The steps leading up to the realization that we have a need to know something are rarely clear, but we do seem to have the knack of somehow knowing what we do know, and knowing what it is that we need to find out. We are able, subconsciously perhaps, to monitor our states of knowledge about such things. This is not to suggest that we are always successful, but only that we succeed frequently enough to make sustained mental activity possible. We may decide to put on a particular sweater before going outdoors and, upon opening a drawer, discover it is not where we thought it was. Infrequent mistakes of this kind can be annoying, but if they happened too often we would scarcely be able to function. When we are quite certain about something and subsequent events prove us to be wrong, we may be surprised or embarrassed, but this is only because our beliefs about the state of our knowledge are usually correct. In addition to knowing about different features of the world, we also have various degrees of confidence in our knowledge. Without bothering to look at them, I have a high degree of confidence in the knowledge that my right hand has five digits, and I would not bother to stop and count them while buying a pair of gloves. I might well do this, however, if my life were at stake over the matter. In contrast, I would no longer place a bet on the accuracy of my knowledge of the foramina through which the cranial nerves pass.

The occasions upon which we recognize a clear need to find out some particular thing are usually those involving a task or performance. We recognize these occasions when we must pause to look up a telephone number, check the proper dose of a drug that we use rarely, or find the normal values for an unfamiliar laboratory test. Our recognition of the need to do such things is automatic and occurs almost subconsciously. When we are absorbed in reflection about some subject, or even during sleep, this monitoring persists. If when traveling we wake up in a strange room, we may momentarily wonder where we are, but we are never in doubt as to who we are. And we are more or less aware of the things that we do not know.[1] How does this come about?

It would seem that our knowledge, especially our propositional knowledge, tends to be clustered about particular topics. Which is only to say that we know more about some subjects than others. Our knowledge of some topics may be solidly anchored to neighboring and closely related established facts, and our attention can rove back and forth among them with confidence. Our knowledge of other topics may form isolated islands which we have not yet succeeded in connecting up. Knowledge of a particular subject seems most thorough and secure at some internal and central point, and as we move out from this central point it becomes more fragmentary, shallower and, at the edges, doubtful. Here, at the borders of a subject matter, we begin to feel uncertain about things.

A suggestion of Belkin's is that we may have what he refers to as "anomalous states of knowledge," by means of which an individual realizes that there is something wrong with his state of knowledge about a particular subject [8]. Belkin suggests that this "wrongness" may be of several kinds. Although we may feel uncomfortable about our state of knowledge regarding something, we can set about correcting matters only after we determine the nature of the "wrongness" involved. Figure 8.1 (after Belkin) provides an example of the case of a well-integrated state of knowledge with one anomalous concept.

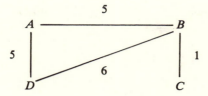

Figure 8.1. An anomalous state of knowledge in which concepts *A, B,* and *D* are well integrated, but the concept *C* is weakly related to only one of the others (after Belkin).

In this diagram, the concepts are indicated by letters, and the numbers represent the strength of the relationships between concepts. The anomaly here is whether the weakly associated concept *C* should in fact be a part of the state of knowledge (*ABD*). Belkin is here using a model somewhat similar to what we have referred to earlier as a "knowledge network." His suggestion is consistent with our belief that if our concepts relate to one another in a coherent and interconnected way, our knowledge is more certain.

Figure 8.2 represents a state of knowledge in which two concepts are questionably related.

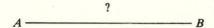

Figure 8.2. A state of knowledge in which two concepts are questionably related (after Belkin).

When this question arises in our minds (whether in fact *A* has anything to do with *B*), we may be moved to inquire further into the details of *A* and *B*.

Another of Belkin's examples is that of a large number of concepts that are weakly related, and with none playing a central role, as suggested in figure 8.3.

His purpose in proposing the concept of an anomalous state of knowledge was to attempt to explain the origin of formal inquiries, such as those required with mechanized information-retrieval systems. Here it is necessary for an inquirer to formulate his inquiry in a form sufficiently precise and unambiguous to enable an information system to act upon it successfully. Belkin implies that

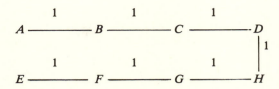

Figure 8.3. A number of concepts that are weakly linked, without a strong central focus (after Belkin).

the first task for the inquirer is to determine his own state of mind regarding the topic in question, and identify the anomalous states of knowledge that may exist in his mind. When it has been determined that there is a need for information, its nature may be more closely specified. A simple case would be that of recognizing the need for some single, well-defined piece of information, such as a telephone number. In this case it would be only knowledge of the number that would be required, and not information about how to use the telephone. We usually do not want *more* information than we need.

We saw examples similar to this when we considered the structure of such questions as: "Where is the post office?" "What is the common logarithm of 2142?" "Where does John Jones live?" These all have the form:

$$(N \| A_1, A_2, A_3, ?, A_4, \ldots)$$

The attributes provided explicitly or through context serve to specify the nominal, and then draw a hearer's attention to the requested attribute. The more carefully we phrase a question, the more likely it is that a forthcoming reply will satisfy our specific need.

It is a common experience to find ourselves unable to formulate a question satisfactorily. We may not know enough about a subject to be able to ask the "right" questions. If this occurs in a library or while interacting with a computerized data base, we may attempt to resolve matters by browsing. By informally or casually scanning materials that are related to the subject of interest we may hope to find clues that will help us sharpen our questions. As we proceed with this process, certain of our states of knowledge may be refreshed or strengthened, and we may find clues to put us on the right track. Information retrieval, whether attempted by what we hope is a formal and focused inquiry, or more casually by browsing, may be an inexact process depending upon the hierarchical level involved. Overall, the process of question formation would appear to involve the following:

1. The inquirer experiences an anomalous state of knowledge.
2. He or she will then attempt to determine more exactly what the anomaly is. Is it the need of a single fact, information to strengthen a hypothesis, a needed small set of information statements, an intact piece of a knowledge network, or an understanding of some entire theory?
3. The nature of the anomaly can then be articulated with reference to content and boundaries, and the inquiry formulated.

The asking of questions involves still another element: the means we have for concluding whether a proffered answer is a satisfactory one. A useful answer might be looked upon as being congruent to a question in much the same way that a piece of a jigsaw puzzle fits into an incompleted portion of the puzzle. The question itself would be a satisfactory one if, by the same analogy, it is congruent to the anomalous state of knowledge experienced by the inquirer. But answers may be satisfactory for unanticipated reasons. With some questions—"What is Dr. Jones's office telephone number?" or "Did Mr. Brown require any pain medication last night?"—what would count as satisfactory answers might seem obvious. Yet there are other responses to these questions that would be equally satisfactory, though unexpected: "Dr. Jones is on vacation in Europe" or "Mr. Brown died early this morning, and we have been trying to reach you." Such nonresponsive replies are not formal answers to our questions, but they may satisfy our reasons for asking them. We commonly reply to a questioner's query in this way, by responding to an evident need or intention rather than to the question itself.

Our anomalous states of knowledge may arise for other reasons: from the circumstance that although we can account for an accident victim's pain in the leg (due to recent trauma) we cannot account for his fever. If we simply ask the question, "Why does this injured patient have fever?" it may not be immediately answerable. So instead of asking such direct or proximate questions, we may circle around the subject and ask indirect ones: "Does the patient have an infection?" "Did the patient receive a blood transfusion while being treated for the injury?'' or ''Did the patient sustain a head injury in the accident?'' Instead of asking unanswerable questions, we will go to some lengths to formulate questions that are answerable, if we think the answers to them might in turn lead us closer to our goal.[2]

Question formation is part of a continuous negotiating process. Whether we are seeking answers from a colleague, a computer-based information system, or from nature, our goal is to remedy an anomalous state of knowledge. A question stemming from a deep-lying concern with universals or general truths is not likely to find a ready answer in clinical medicine. Faced with a cancer patient in the consulting room, the physician does not idly speculate on the causes of cancer. Instead he will ask himself potentially answerable questions, such as ''How certain am I of the diagnosis?'' ''How can I determine the present extent of the disease?'' and always, ''How best can I help this patient?''

Analyzing the process of question formation is difficult because of the well-recognized shortcomings of introspection. Examining a patient, asking questions, and entertaining several diagnostic possibilities all at the same time involves so much cognitive activity that its subsequent analysis may be impossible. Elstein has reviewed in detail the techniques that have been used in attempting to analyze these activities as they arise during medical diagnosis. Yet, despite such efforts, the processes by means of which we are prompted to formulate clinical questions remains unclear. A quite different approach to the study of question formation may become possible as a result of work with so-called question-answering or expert systems. This is a broad field of activity, but one aspect of it is pertinent to the present discussion.

A research project of Martin Epstein's exemplifies these possibilities. Epstein's project involved the assembly of a data base containing clinical data obtained from patients who had been cared for in our Melanoma Clinic. In order to facilitate the use of this data base by clinicians, a so-called natural language front end was developed. This type of interactive program makes it possible to make inquiries of a data base by means of questions expressed in natural language, and avoids the need for a user to learn a special query or procedural language or, alternatively, of employing a programmer as an intermediary. In this project, a number of patient records had been entered into the system. Each patient's initial clinical state and subsequent course were described by using up to 150 different clinical attributes. The nature of the task domain and the types of data in the system made it a point B undertaking, in the terminology of the previous chapter.

One of the issues that arose early in the course of this project was, What kinds of questions might users wish to ask? This question is one that every designer of a data-base system must ask (whether it involves natural-language inquiry or not), and especially so if it is intended to serve as a "question-answering" or "expert" system. This turns out to be a surprisingly difficult question to answer. It is easy enough to compose a list of "typical" questions and assume that if the system can process them it could presumably answer questions that would be asked by its eventual users. But I have personally found in attempting to create such questions that, although they might adequately test the system and could well be the kinds of questions that physicians would actually ask, there always seemed to be something artificial about them. The questions most easily posed always seemed to be contrived and uninteresting ones. Beyond this, I usually experienced a feeling of frustration in attempting to create such questions. When Epstein's experimental system became operable, I began to understand why this had been so. We ordinarily do not create questions in response to a request to do so; they arise spontaneously in concrete situations. And though questions come into mind naturally in these particular situations, it is with a curious and even uncomfortable feeling that we attempt to create them in the abstract.[3]

My experiences in using Epstein's program suggests that they may be relevant to the general subject of browsing. In using his rapid and convenient interactive system, I soon experienced the following as I began to explore the data base. After asking some rather contrived questions to get things started (and being provided in return with certain data or lists, which were really not of much interest), further questions concerning these results would spontaneously come to mind. These questions were then asked of the system, and the answers the next time around tended to be more interesting. These in turn prompted still further questions, which were then explored. This dynamic interaction itself soon began to create contexts, and suggested other questions that had been far from my mind at the start. After a few such cycles, it became clear that although my earlier questions had been far from insightful, they were getting better and I was even beginning to ask the "right" questions. Only then did it occur to me that I was not only exploring the data base but also using it as a tool to explore my own state of knowledge and concepts regarding melanoma. And this exploration was not a trivial testing of my own store of simple facts, but the much more fascinating exploration of how the creation of questions and hypotheses is stimulated, producing some questions and hypotheses of considerable interest which had simply not occurred to me before.

Some years ago our melanoma group, together with those of three other medical centers, had joined in a cooperative clinical study of melanoma and had accumulated a large amount of standardized information concerning more than 1,000 carefully studied new melanoma patients. These clinical data had been stored in a computer-based system that had not been provided with a general retrieval capability (these not being available at the time). Although individual patient records could be easily retrieved, the aggregation of particular attributes *across* the entire set of patients was carried out only with difficulty. Each inquiry required the writing of a small program, and thus necessitated the interposition of a programmer between the clinician (who is most likely to formulate insightful questions) and the data. The potential usefulness of these data could not, therefore, be readily realized. One cannot browse in such a data base, and the clinical investigators who had participated in the collection of the data were deprived of the convenience and stimulation provided by an interactive system.

These experiences are consistent with quite general principles. If our questions result in a prompt response (feedback), we profit from this to a degree that delayed responses wholly fail to achieve. Although some of our ideas or questions may be persistent ones, and our interest in them sustained over long periods of time, many are fleeting. Our attention span at certain levels of detail may be unfortunately short. If it requires a substantial effort (or expense or delay) to obtain answers to certain of our questions, we may not bother with them or persist in our search for answers. It is in facilitating this inquiry or discovery process that we can expect interactive data bases and question-answering systems to prove of great value in medicine.

In addition to supporting the process of search and discovery, these systems may contribute to the understanding of the question-forming process itself. This may be a reasonable expectation for several reasons. When computer systems like the one described are used, the inquiry process becomes both more formal and more serial than is the case when using other information sources. A record of attempted retrievals can easily be kept by the program, and if at some later time we may wonder how our inquiry proceeded in a particular instance, access to such records would be extremely revealing. It would simplify attempts at introspection and improve the use of "protocols," especially in comparison with a situation in which several channels of perception are operating simultaneously, or when cognitive processing occurs in parallel.

All these matters relate to our efforts to ascertain our anomalous states of knowledge. Only when this is completed can we articulate the questions that accurately reflect our needs. When questions are being asked in a dialogue with a human consultant or with an interactive computer system, we are able continuously to revise our questions depending on the previous responses. The great advantage of interacting with a human expert or teacher is that during this process it is possible (and common) for the expert to recognize just what it is that the questioner needs to know and to point it out. The advantage of the computer system is that it can hold extremely large amounts of raw and organized data and thus be capable, through suitable questioning, of providing answers known to no one.

The "questioner-expert" designation applies to most of us since each of us is either a "questioner" or an "expert" for a part of the time. As questioners (if left to our own resources) we can only extend our knowledge of things by building upon what we already know in incremental steps. A teacher or consultant may be able to spot our difficulty and point us to a shortcut or refer us to a theory or to a body of knowledge of which we had been unaware. But the reason he is able to recognize our needs is because our question-answer dialogues occur in shared human situations. Because of this, it seems unlikely that "question-answering" systems or "teaching-machines" will ever reach the level of imaginative helpfulness that a human expert or teacher can provide. Nevertheless, the ability of knowledge-based "question-answering systems" to supply answers to queries regarding newly acquired or incompletely organized experimental (clinical) data may be of particular promise. This ability could assist in the creation of new information which no human expert could be expected to provide. Clinical data-base systems, with their data-management capabilities and their interactive probing should greatly increase the rate of discovery, and become increasingly effective in the creation of new medical knowledge.

8.2 Words As Keys

Common objects have been so frequently observed and talked about that their most distinctive attributes are all named, and knowing these names is a part of our ordinary knowledge of the world. We know that butter can have the attributes "fresh" or "rancid," but that milk is "fresh" or "sour." These usages are so well known to us that upon hearing the isolated word *rancid,* we might think of butter or vegetable oil, but we would not think of milk. To a physician, the medical words that are used to name clinical objects and attributes appear to direct his reasoning in a similar way. Technical terms may thus act as keys which selectively point to categories or classes of things, and sometimes even to single things, such as a particular disease. Words vary greatly in their ability to do this.

Suppose someone were to take his automobile into a garage with the complaint that it made a "funny noise." This would provide a mechanic with relatively little information. A more articulate car owner might use the word "rattle." To the mechanic this would call to mind certain kinds of causes. A "rattle" is a particular kind of noise, and when this word is used correctly it is more specific and it conveys more information. But if a still more knowledgeable driver were to tell the mechanic that the car had a "knock," that would be much more specific and the mechanic would probably be led to a quick diagnosis of the problem.

In considering the connections between words and their designated objects (their referents), we are speaking of the mappings between objects or classes of objects in the actual world and the symbols we use in referring to them. The words we use in referring to lower-level objects seem to map one-to-one, and those referring to higher-level things tend to map one-to-many. The word *electron* has no synonyms and needs none; the word *house* has many, and we need them all. We succeed in designating particular high-level objects by the use of proper names, but these work only within suitable contexts. "John" may be a unique designator when employed in a family setting, but in a classroom the use of "John Smith" might be required. In a larger group (or to identify a particular patient's medical record) even "John Smith" would be insufficient, and we would need further particulars, such as date of birth or Social Security number.

These symbols, which we use to construct our models of reality, occur in a number of forms, but those of greatest interest to us here are words. We must have the answers to two questions concerning medical words in order to find their two relevant properties: "What is the specificity of a given word for a particular object, and how is this affected by its hierarchical level?" And, second, "Are the relationships occurring among these objects (the structure of the world) reflected in the relationships we find among the corresponding words?"

We will first consider the matter of selectivity—the degree to which words point to particular things. This selective property of words is one that is much used as we talk or reason about things in medicine. Let us explore some of the semantic properties of "medical words" and the selectivity that these terms have with respect to categories of disease or to diseases themselves. For this purpose

Colorado Tick Fever 00 2217

AT	Fever, mountain; fever, mountain tick.
ET	Virus transmitted by tick Dermancentor andersoni.
SM	Chills; headache; photophobia; backache; pain in eye; myalgia; anorexia; nausea; vomiting; prostration.
SG	Seasonal, March to July, in western United States; incubation period 4-6 days; onset abrupt; possibly slight erythema; sustained fever, 102°-104°F or higher significant; pulse rate increased. Course: In prevention, removal of tick from skin; applications to skin of turpentine, iodine, acetone; removal of tick by insertion of needle between mouth parts; aspirin for pain; antibiotic treatment ineffective.
CM	Encephalitis, meningitis especially in children.
LB	WBC decreased: monocytosis; complement-fixation test positive; injection of serum of CSF killing suckling mice; neutralization of virus with immune serum resulting in survival.

Figure 8.4. The description of Colorado tick fever in *Current Medical Information and Terminology* (CMIT) (Chicago: American Medical Association, 1971) (with permission of the A.M.A.).

we will draw upon some experimental results obtained from studies with CMIT, the compendium of diseases described earlier. The text of this book is highly structured, and most of the information is provided in the form of single words and phrases. It will be noted (see fig. 8.4) that the style and syntax are unconventional, and that the disease descriptions are essentially in $(N \| A)$ form. In such a telegraphic style complete sentences occur only rarely, although the text is readily understood. The information is conveyed largely by the semantic properties of the medical terms used, and the indicated context.

Some diseases reflect disturbances of particular body systems, whereas others involve several systems or even the body as a whole. Most disease classification schemes take this into account. CMIT does this by assigning diseases to the following conventional categories:

Category	
00	Body as a whole, including psyche
01	Skin
02	Musculoskeletal
03	Respiratory
04	Cardiovascular
05	Blood and lymphatic
06	Digestive
07	Genitourinary
08	Endocrine
09	Nervous
10	Organs of special sense

The authors of CMIT, in addition to describing each disease, assigned each disease to one of these categories, as appropriate, or to two at most. Such assignments are arbitrary, but they seem reasonable enough given the degree of abstraction involved. As an example, metabolic acidosis has been assigned to category 00, and respiratory acidosis to 03. A disorder such as herpangina (hand, foot, and mouth disease), which necessarily involves the skin *and* oral mucosa, is assigned to 01 and 06, whereas lichen planus, which ordinarily involves the skin and less commonly the mouth, is assigned to 01. Such an allocation of diseases to body systems is a conventional, if not an entirely unambiguous, procedure. This

3206 of	507 small	364 other
2865 in	492 possible	360 acute
2405 possibly	489 severe	360 years
2315 with	478 most	358 failure
2104 course	473 disease	349 between
2010 to	457 pressure	349 large
1953 or	447 absence	341 dyspnea
1408 by	446 trauma	341 early
1379 usually	443 chronic	340 weakness
1194 pain	442 edema	339 nausea
980 as	435 percent	338 tenderness
945 on	434 treatment	337 inflammation
889 from	432 vomiting	337 mass
812 infection	431 later	336 age
766 features	426 absent	335 within
749 unknown	422 common	332 if
738 at	421 asymptomatic	331 lower
716 cells	420 during	328 swelling
699 associated	415 rarely	327 necrosis
682 increased	414 hereditary	325 positive
674 onset	401 lesions	324 headache
666 tissue	396 than	318 frequent
650 blood	390 abdominal	316 wbc
627 normal	389 more	315 area
619 skin	389 often	313 hemorrhage
603 and	383 into	313 infiltration
596 for	382 type	309 obstruction
575 rare	381 bone	304 from
553 fever	375 involvement	301 congenital
541 loss	369 especially	301 enlargement
538 after	367 areas	301 progressive

Figure 8.5. Most commonly used words in CMIT; the prefixed number is the number of disease descriptions in which the given word occurs at least once.

crude division of diseases serves many practical ends, and it is sanctioned by the naming of the clinical specialties. The first question, then, is the extent to which the semantics of the medical terms employed in CMIT for describing diseases connote specific organ systems or categories of disease.

The vocabulary used in CMIT consists of 21,415 different words,[4] of which the most frequently used are the common words *of, in,* and *possibly.*[5] Figure 8.5 lists the most often used of these common words. The disease attribute most frequently employed in CMIT is "pain," which occurs in the descriptions of 1,194 different diseases (out of a total of 3,262). For a patient to complain of pain in some general manner could do no more than direct a physician's attention to those 1,194 "painful" diseases. This attribute therefore has what we will term a low "selection power."[6] A symptom or sign that occurred in *all* diseases would have no selectivity whatever. In contrast, a pathognomonic (sufficient) attribute would have a maximal selectivity, and would point unmistakably to a single disease. The medical terms that stand for disease attributes (clinical or laboratory findings) can therefore be assigned selectivities which, in our study, were assigned values ranging between zero and one. They will tend to direct our attention either to a particular disease or to a disease category with a corresponding degree of likelihood. This property of medical terms figures prominently in diagnosis.

For our estimate of "selectivity," we computed for each of the 21,415 words in CMIT the number of different disease descriptions in which each word occurred at least once. We then took the reciprocal of this number and normalized it to the unit interval.[7] Under this procedure, a word that was uniquely associated with a single disease (such as *Koplik* with *measles*) would have a selectivity of nearly one, whereas a word that was used in the descriptions of all diseases (the word *of* has the highest frequency, appearing in 3,208 out of the 3,262 disease descriptions) would have a selectivity of zero.

In examining CMIT, it was evident that some of the words were medical terms (e.g., *dysuria*) and others were ordinary words commonly used in everyday language, which could not be expected to have any particular relation to diseases. An overall word frequency study of CMIT showed (expectedly) that the most commonly used words were for the most part "ordinary English words'' (fig. 8.5). This frequency count also showed that slightly over half the words used occurred only once, and that those were a mixture of uncommon medical terms having very specific meanings and common English words that were in no way remarkable. These latter words, though occurring rarely and thus having a formally high selectivity, should in fact be assigned none at all. The question, then, was how one might go about separating the "medical terms" from the "common English words." The prospect of going through this vocabulary of 21,415 words, one at a time, and making that many individual judgments was not appealing. More serious was the fact that we had no basis or theory for making such judgments at all. Is *blood* a medical term or a common English word? It is clearly both. Instead of forcing our interpretation upon such matters, we decided to explore the question experimentally and see how the CMIT authors had actually employed these words.

We approached this by reasoning in the following way. A common word such as *of* is a general-purpose lexical tool, which we can use (and may need) in speaking about anything. A medical term such as *dysuria* has a much narrower range of application. Although it points to no particular disease, it calls to mind a particular class of diseases, certain disorders of the genitourinary system. Since the diseases in CMIT had been assigned to particular physiological systems, it appeared that we might be able to define a measure for the semantic span of individual words. For each word in CMIT that occurred more than once we counted the number of occurrences in each of the eleven disease categories, which resulted in a set of eleven numbers that could be thought of as a vector of eleven components. A specific medical term like *dysuria* would be expected to occur most frequently in the category "genitourinary" (07), although it might occur in a few other categories. A common English word such as *of*, in contrast, would be expected to show no association with any particular disease category, and therefore to occur with comparable frequencies in all of them.

In order to measure the selective power, we defined an "entropy-like" function computed over the vector components. This was done in a conventional way so that a word which occurred in only one disease category would have a low entropy. For words occurring in only one category, those with the greater number of occurrences would have the lesser entropy.[8] A program was written to compute these measures (the vector components and the entropies), and they were then calculated for all the words in CMIT that occurred more than once. The words were then sorted in increasing order of entropy. Figure 8.6 shows the low-entropy end (top) of this list, and figure 8.7 shows the terms at the high-entropy end. At the top of the first list we find the entries *lens, cornea,* and "pbi." The two words are used in describing eyes and their diseases (organs of special sense, category 10), and the third entry is the common abbreviation for a particular laboratory test (protein-bound iodine) specifically related to thyroid function (the endocrine system, category 08). The words occurring at the bottom of the entropy list (the highest entropy words) are just those common English words that we would have expected to find here. This algorithmic procedure therefore provides us with a means for beginning to separate the medical terms from the common English words. An examination of this overall entropy list (which consists of approximately 9,000 words) showed that the top third consisted of medical terms, the bottom third of nonmedical terms ("ordinary" English words), and the middle third contained a mixture of the two. What we had been seeking was a measure of the specificity of the medical words used for disease attributes, and we were now able to proceed with this by focusing our attention upon the words in the top third of this list.

One of our hopes in studying the selectivity of medical words was to determine whether medical knowledge represented in the form employed in CMIT might be used in a computer program intended for the generation of differential diagnoses. Donald Lindberg's early work on the CONSIDER program, which was the first to employ CMIT for this purpose, was designed to utilize entered disease attributes, and to search for diseases in which the attributes occurred in stipulated Boolean combinations. CONSIDER employed a series of inverted word files and pointers, which offered great economies in processing compared with a direct searching of the CMIT text. Our initial experimental work with CMIT was begun at this level of performance. It quickly became apparent to us, as it had to Lindberg and his colleagues earlier, that this approach had severe limitations. First, the search procedure required an exact lexical match. If the plural term *pains* were entered, it would not match *pain* in a disease description.

0.8762	.02	.02	.02	.02	.01	.02	.01	.01	.03	.02	.83	lens	50
1.0204	.05	.04	.01	.02	.02	.03	.02	.00	.02	.01	.77	cornea	79
1.0278	.02	.01	.02	.02	.04	.04	.02	.01	.78	.02	.03	pbi	18
1.0369	.04	.01	.01	.77	.04	.02	.01	.01	.03	.04	.02	expectoration	54
1.0377	.02	.01	.03	.01	.74	.11	.02	.01	.02	.01	.02	murmur	86
1.0411	.03	.01	.01	.02	.77	.03	.02	.01	.04	.02	.03	atrium	45
1.0422	.04	.01	.01	.02	.02	.03	.02	.01	.04	.03	.77	ciliary	33
1.0658	.03	.04	.02	.02	.02	.02	.01	.01	.03	.03	.76	iris	53
1.0667	.01	.01	.01	.02	.03	.03	.03	.01	.76	.02	.05	uptake	20
1.0885	.05	.01	.01	.02	.03	.03	.01	.02	.76	.03	.02	iodine	27
1.1236	.08	.01	.01	.03	.02	.74	.03	.01	.03	.01	.03	hemoglobin	51
1.1298	.01	.01	.02	.05	.74	.04	.02	.02	.05	.02	.03	qrs	41
1.1361	.02	.01	.02	.01	.69	.16	.02	.02	.02	.01	.01	systolic	91
1.1465	.03	.03	.03	.02	.02	.02	.02	.01	.03	.04	.74	glaucoma	49
1.1504	.07	.01	.01	.72	.09	.02	.02	.02	.02	.01	.01	rales	96
1.1556	.05	.00	.02	.05	.70	.01	.01	.01	.12	.02	.01	ecg	150
1.1642	.01	.02	.02	.73	.04	.04	.02	.01	.05	.02	.03	bronchoscopy	26
1.1716	.07	.02	.06	.02	.01	.02	.01	.01	.03	.02	.72	cataract	53
1.1812	.02	.03	.01	.03	.04	.04	.01	.01	.03	.07	.72	retina	61
1.1959	.01	.03	.03	.03	.02	.04	.02	.73	.05	.02	.03	urethral	64
1.2069	.01	.03	.02	.03	.02	.04	.02	.72	.05	.02	.03	urethra	52
1.2106	.01	.02	.02	.03	.02	.04	.02	.72	.06	.02	.04	cystoscopy	53
1.2124	.03	.02	.02	.03	.02	.04	.02	.01	.05	.04	.72	vitreous	24
1.2262	.02	.70	.01	.02	.02	.02	.02	.08	.03	.01	.06	epidermis	93
1.2293	.03	.01	.02	.03	.04	.04	.02	.72	.05	.02	.03	cervix	64
1.2493	.06	.01	.03	.02	.70	.05	.01	.01	.06	.03	.02	atrial	65
1.2551	.05	.01	.02	.02	.04	.01	.01	.01	.06	.08	.69	vision	192
1.2560	.02	.03	.02	.03	.04	.04	.02	.01	.05	.02	.71	intraocular	23
1.2583	.04	.01	.02	.05	.02	.04	.02	.70	.05	.02	.03	pyuria	65
1.2689	.04	.01	.04	.04	.01	.05	.01	.69	.07	.01	.02	uterus	96
1.2758	.01	.02	.02	.06	.69	.05	.02	.01	.06	.02	.04	angiocardiography	30
1.2913	.01	.01	.02	.05	.64	.03	.01	.01	.07	.14	.01	ventricle	95
1.3008	.01	.04	.02	.05	.04	.04	.03	.03	.69	.02	.03	adenoma	21
1.3089	.01	.68	.02	.02	.01	.02	.06	.04	.06	.04	.04	dermis	85
1.3092	.01	.03	.04	.02	.02	.05	.03	.07	.69	.03	.02	hormone	44
1.3108	.09	.01	.01	.67	.03	.03	.05	.02	.06	.01	.02	sputum	57
1.3120	.02	.01	.02	.08	.67	.07	.02	.01	.05	.02	.03	mitral	38
1.3176	.05	.01	.03	.02	.04	.08	.02	.68	.03	.01	.02	uterine	98
1.3185	.04	.02	.02	.69	.02	.05	.02	.03	.06	.02	.04	alveoli	24
1.3190	.03	.06	.02	.01	.01	.02	.02	.07	.68	.03	.05	pituitary	52
1.3211	.03	.03	.01	.05	.67	.05	.01	.01	.07	.04	.02	aorta	60
1.3224	.05	.06	.03	.02	.04	.68	.02	.01	.05	.02	.03	splenectomy	27
1.3269	.02	.02	.02	.04	.03	.68	.03	.02	.07	.03	.05	target	11
1.3317	.02	.03	.04	.04	.04	.03	.04	.69	.04	.01	.02	vaginal	91
1.3344	.03	.02	.02	.03	.08	.05	.02	.03	.06	.02	.04	gallop	29
1.3369	.03	.02	.01	.06	.10	.03	.03	.01	.04	.01	.66	chamber	41
1.3375	.05	.02	.02	.03	.04	.04	.02	.02	.68	.02	.07	hyperglycemia	18

1.3378	.04	.03	.03	.04	.02	.02	.01	.00	.05	.08	.67	eye	113
1.3395	.04	.01	.01	.06	.65	.05	.01	.01	.06	.07	.01	ventricular	110
1.3439	.02	.03	.02	.02	.02	.04	.02	.01	.05	.13	.65	pupil	29
1.3560	.15	.03	.01	.01	.01	.02	.01	.01	.07	.08	.61	corneal	84
1.3585	.02	.02	.02	.02	.03	.15	.01	.04	.64	.02	.62	bmr	28
1.3605	.02	.02	.02	.03	.65	.12	.04	.01	.05	.02	.03	valve	35

Figure 8.6. List of the lowest entropy words in CMIT. The first column is the entropy calculated by the formula given in the footnote. The next 11 columns give the number of diseases in which the word occurs (expressed as a percent) in each of the 11 disease categories, listed in conventional order. The right-most number is the total number of diseases in which the word occurs at least once. Thus, the word *lens* is used in 50 different disease descriptions, and 83 percent of these diseases are in the category "organs of special sense."

2.3626	.08	.05	.08	.11	.13	.07	.08	.10	.11	.07	.08	degree	124
2.3629	.08	.06	.05	.09	.14	.13	.05	.07	.11	.09	.09	absent	426
2.3639	.09	.12	.09	.07	.11	.10	.05	.06	.13	.11	.18	blotchy	8
2.3635	.05	.09	.11	.07	.10	.07	.10	.10	.13	.11	.07	common	422
2.3637	.12	.08	.09	.07	.05	.11	.10	.10	.14	.05	.09	china	8
2.3640	.10	.10	.10	.09	.10	.09	.09	.09	.05	.14	.06	within	335
2.3642	.18	.11	.12	.09	.08	.19	.13	.10	.06	.09	.05	marked	159
2.3647	.11	.08	.11	.04	.07	.13	.09	.08	.08	.10	.11	indicative	20
2.3653	.07	.09	.12	.05	.12	.09	.07	.10	.07	.11	.11	absence	447
2.3660	.09	.04	.08	.07	.09	.11	.09	.10	.09	.13	.12	milder	44
2.3667	.12	.06	.08	.13	.11	.07	.09	.10	.09	.06	.09	week	45
2.3668	.07	.09	.08	.06	.13	.10	.11	.10	.11	.09	.06	often	389
2.3678	.11	.05	.09	.10	.09	.07	.07	.11	.13	.07	.11	simple	46
2.3681	.12	.11	.06	.09	.08	.09	.07	.07	.14	.08	.09	2	130
2.3687	.09	.09	.09	.10	.08	.08	.09	.14	.12	.05	.07	large	349
2.3701	.08	.07	.13	.09	.13	.06	.09	.10	.07	.07	.11	causing	256
2.3708	.10	.06	.10	.10	.10	.14	.10	.06	.07	.09	.07	severe	489
2.3711	.06	.06	.02	.02	.10	.09	.11	.07	.11	.09	.09	late	125
2.3716	.09	.10	.11	.05	.13	.09	.08	.08	.06	.10	.11	without	246
2.3718	.09	.08	.08	.08	.11	.09	.13	.12	.09	.09	.05	if	332
2.3718	.10	.09	.09	.08	.13	.10	.09	.05	.11	.07	.09	increasing	123
2.3724	.13	.10	.10	.10	.05	.09	.07	.08	.11	.08	.09	for	596
2.3727	.07	.07	.13	.07	.11	.12	.08	.08	.11	.09	.08	than	396
2.3746	.06	.11	.10	.18	.08	.10	.11	.11	.08	.11	.06	most	478
2.3746	.07	.12	.13	.07	.10	.10	.10	.09	.06	.08	.08	each	30
2.3746	.09	.08	.09	.09	.07	.10	.08	.16	.11	.13	.09	onset	674
2.3748	.11	.09	.07	.08	.07	.11	.08	.08	.07	.10	.14	accumulation	61
2.3762	.09	.10	.07	.08	.11	.12	.07	.06	.11	.11	.07	poor	55
2.3776	.07	.11	.14	.08	.08	.09	.08	.08	.11	.10	.07	more	389
2.3780	.10	.09	.12	.05	.08	.10	.07	.09	.10	.11	.09	and	693

2.3792	.16	.09	.09	.10	.06	.11	.10	.09	.12	.09	.10	type 382
2.3793	.06	.09	.08	.07	.10	.10	.09	.10	.13	.09	.08	rarely 415
2.3794	.08	.08	.08	.08	.08	.12	.12	.10	.09	.11	.07	variable 205
2.3794	.09	.08	.08	.10	.12	.08	.09	.08	.08	.13	.08	cases 260
2.3801	.09	.09	.10	.07	.09	.12	.10	.12	.07	.08	.07	frequent 318
2.3815	.06	.10	.08	.11	.09	.08	.07	.08	.11	.11	.11	later 431
2.3819	.08	.08	.10	.11	.12	.09	.08	.10	.10	.09	.06	during 420
2.3821	.07	.10	.10	.11	.11	.08	.10	.06	.10	.09	.08	especially 369
2.3847	.06	.11	.11	.08	.09	.08	.09	.11	.08	.10	.10	usually 1379
2.3847	.12	.10	.07	.10	.07	.07	.09	.09	.09	.11	.09	general 78
2.3855	.11	.09	.09	.09	.09	.09	.07	.07	.08	.09	.12	as 980
2.3863	.08	.10	.10	.09	.08	.08	.10	.10	.07	.09	.12	of 3209
2.3888	.09	.09	.08	.08	.09	.10	.08	.11	.07	.08	.11	from 889
2.3892	.09	.09	.08	.08	.07	.10	.11	.09	.11	.07	.10	after 538
2.3899	.08	.11	.10	.08	.09	.08	.10	.10	.08	.08	.11	with 2315
2.3902	.09	.09	.09	.08	.09	.10	.08	.10	.07	.09	.12	early 341
2.3911	.08	.11	.10	.08	.08	.08	.10	.10	.08	.09	.11	in 2865
2.3914	.09	.11	.09	.08	.08	.09	.09	.10	.09	.08	.11	by 1408
2.3919	.09	.11	.09	.08	.08	.10	.08	.09	.08	.09	.11	coarse 2104
2.3986	.07	.10	.10	.08	.10	.09	.10	.10	.08	.09	.10	or 1953
2.3950	.08	.10	.10	.09	.09	.08	.09	.10	.09	.09	.10	possibly 2405
2.3955	.08	.10	.10	.09	.09	.08	.09	.09	.08	.09	.10	to 2010

Figure 8.7. List of the highest entropy words in CMIT. (See caption for fig. 8.6.) The highest entropy word, *to,* is seen to occur with nearly equal frequency in all disease categories.

Next, the matter of synonymy raised further problems. Entering the term *pruritus* would not retrieve a disease in which the synonym *itch* were used, or vice versa. Third, the process of negation raised still other difficulties. Entering the term *pain* would produce a match with a disease in which the phrase *without pain* occurred.

The result of requiring an exact match led to the conclusion that these programs could utilize only a few attributes, and this was particularly evident when they were connected with the Boolean "and." It was found that if two disease attributes generated a list of, say, fifty diseases in which both terms appeared, adding a third attribute might reduce this to twenty, but that adding a fourth revealed that there was no disease in which they all occurred. The Boolean "and" was simply too strong a logical condition. The program was thus intolerant of the contingent nature of many disease attributes, and in a logic sense it was far too "hard edged." This was disappointing, if predictable, because, from an informational point of view, the performance of diagnostic programs should improve as greater amounts of information are provided it.

When it had been shown that the "selectivity" of attributes could be computed, a new program was written that used this measure. The selection power of each word in CMIT was then calculated according to the formula $S = (1 - n/3262)$, cited earlier, and stored. A set of clinical attributes could then be entered, one at a time, to retrieve all the diseases in which they occurred, and the implicated diseases placed on a list. A score was assigned to each disease equal to the sum of the selectivities of the terms used in producing the match. As additional terms were entered, diseases were added to the list, and their individual scores were accumulated. When the search and scoring process was completed, the diseases were sorted in the order of their accumulated scores. A disease containing all the entered terms would attain the maximum possible score, and appear at the top of the list. In our experience with the program, few diseases attained the maximum score. This happened for several reasons including the matter of synonymy, and the fact that some of the entered terms, though being attributes that a patient with the disease might have, were not included in the CMIT description. This program, however, was able to utilize as many attributes as one wished to enter, and generated disease lists from which reasonable differential diagnoses could be formed. This program was named RECONSIDER, and its performance will be examined shortly.[9]

The RECONSIDER program contained features that made it useful as a research tool. For example, the entered terms could be prefixed by "all" or by a specific "part" (i.e., under "symptoms," "sign," "laboratory," etc.) and the search would then be conducted over the entire disease description, or limited to the designated part. Another feature was a program routine that computed the number of occurrences of an entered term with respect to the eleven disease categories. This permitted us to compute the specificity of a particular disease attribute for each disease *category* as described earlier, and to do this for arbitrary sets of attributes as well. During diagnosis, physicians frequently attempt to infer which physiological systems are involved before they take the next step of choosing a particular disease which is known to affect that system.

Operating as described (but with no steps having been taken

with respect to the issues of synonymy or negation), the program performed surprisingly well. The disease lists generated seemed, for the most part, to be appropriate ones. One way of evaluating the program's performance was to compare it with other diagnostic programs. It must be remembered, however, that these other programs have generally had quite different objectives. Lindberg's CONSIDER program was written to serve a prompting function, to provide a user with a list of possible diseases which a patient with the given attributes might have. RECONSIDER continues in this tradition, and proposes only to generate a list of diseases in which a differential diagnosis is embedded.

Diagnostic programs that seek a single, correct diagnosis are in general much more powerful and correspondingly complex. The CADUCEUS (formerly INTERNIST) program of H. E. Pople and J. D. Myers [84] is the most ambitious of these at present, and attempts to select the correct diagnosis among some 500 or so medical diseases. A program having more restricted aims is one described earlier by Pauker and associates [93], which deals with a set of twenty diseases, all of which are associated with the clinical finding of edema. The performance of these two programs had been described in the literature in sufficient detail to enable us to run their test cases using RECONSIDER.

The program of Pauker et al. (Present Illness Program, or PIP) employs a number of AI techniques (as does CADUCEUS), and it can use both positive and negative findings. Since our program did not have the latter capability, we could use only the positive findings used in their test cases. In their first case, they used approximately forty attributes in their program. Many of these were negative, and others were facts taken from patient histories, which were given special and predefined meanings in their program (e.g., "the patient has small policy life insurance"). For these reasons we could use only nine of the forty listed attributes from this case, all of which represented positive signs or laboratory findings. Figure 8.8 shows the response of our program when these terms were entered.[10] Pauker's second, third, and fourth cases were run in a similar manner, and RECONSIDER's differential diagnoses are compared with PIP's in figure 8.9. The purpose in comparing these results is not to make any performance claims, but to contrast the two very different concepts underlying these programs.

Pauker's program contains a large amount of prestored knowledge about the diseases that may cause edema, about the clinical findings which these diseases may display (together with the conditional probabilities involved), and it provides an appropriate logic to be used in drawing inferences from combinations of these findings. The development of this program required that expert physicians supply this medical knowledge. Our program employed rather different kinds of components: (1) the book CMIT, which contained only a small fraction of the total knowledge of the diseases, and which had been prepared for totally different purposes, (2) a model of disease descriptions (the [$N \parallel A$] model) which suggested the use of certain procedures for measuring similarity, and (3) the concept of the semantic selection power of medical terms. The other major difference between the programs was that ours conducted its search among more than 3,000 different diseases, whereas the edema program made its selection from twenty.

A case that was successfully processed by CADUCEUS has been described in considerable detail by Myers [89]. It was the case of a young male patient with a number of findings suggestive of both

Terms entered into RECONSIDER

pitted, selectivity = 0.989
edema, selectivity = 0.685
periorbital edema, selectivity = 0.997
proteinuria, selectivity = 0.968
albumin, selectivity = 0.977
weight gain, selectivity = 0.988

	5.604	— maximum total score		590 diseases
1	3.620	nephrotic syndrome	07	
2	2.670	hypothyroidism, iodide	08	
3	2.650	hemorrhagic fever, epidemic	00	
4	2.641	preeclampsia	07	
5	2.631	glomerulonephritis, chronic	07	

Figure 8.8. RECONSIDER's computed disease list (top five diseases only) for the entered terms: *pitted, edema, periorbital edema, proteinuria, albumin,* and *weight gain.* The diagnoses obtained by PIP (see text) were: (1) idiopathic nephrotic syndrome (2) acute glomerulonephritis (3) Hennoch-Schoenlein purpura.

Terms entered into RECONSIDER

pedal edema, selectivity = 0.999
pitting, selectivity = 0.996
alcohol, selectivity = 0.971
jaundice, selectivity = 0.906
hepatomegaly, selectivity = 0.929
splenomegaly, selectivity = 0.919
ascites, selectivity = 0.958
palmar erythema, selectivity = 0.999
spider angiomata, selectivity = 1.000
bilirubin, selectivity = 0.974
prothrombin, selectivity = 0.986
sgpt, selectivity = 0.993
sgot, selectivity = 0.983
ldh, selectivity = 0.988
melena, selectivity = 0.979
serum iron, selectivity = 0.997
varices, selectivity = 0.980

	16.557	— maximum total scores	428 diseases
1	6.726	liver, cirrhosis, portal 06	
2	6.713	liver, cirrhosis, postnecrotic 06	
3	6.687	liver, cirrhosis, primary biliary 06	
4	5.703	hepatitis, viral, acute 06	
5	5.688	heart, failure, congestive 04	
6	5.688	hepatitis, lupoid 06	
7	5.671	splenomegaly, congestive chronic 05	
8	5.671	schistosomiasis, mansoni 06	
9	4.799	hepatitis, chemical-induced toxicity 06	
10	4.769	liver, fatty 06	
11	4.765	schistosomiasis, japonica 06	
12	4.750	liver, cirrhosis, with passive congestion 06	
13	4.745	liver, massive necrosis 06	

PIP's diagnoses   FIT:

		FIT:
1.	cirrhosis	0.72
2.	hepatitis	0.75
3.	portal hypertension	0.72
4.	constrictive pericarditis	0.17

Figure 8.9*a, b, c.* RECONSIDER's computed disease list, compared with PIP's results.

Terms entered into RECONSIDER

casts, selectivity = 0.973
toxins, selectivity = 0.993
oliguria, selectivity = 0.979
sodium, selectivity = 0.963
pedal edema, selectivity = 0.999
pitting, selectivity = 0.996

	5.903	— maximum total score	144 diseases
1	2.945	crush syndrome 07	
2	2.915	kidney, failure, acute 07	
3	2.915	nephrocalcinosis 07	
4	2.915	kidney, tubular necrosis, acute 07	
5	1.972	mushroom, toxicity 00	
6	1.972	hepatorenal syndrome 06-07	
7	1.952	carbon tetrachloride, toxicity 00	
8	1.952	heart, hypertensive disease 04	
9	1.952	heart, failure, congestive 04	
10	1.952	kidney, cortex, necrosis 07	

PIP's diagnoses   FIT:

1.	acute tubular necrosis	0.50
2.	acute glomerulonephritis	0.20
3.	idiopathic nephrotic syndrome	0.18
4.	chronic glomerulonephritis	0.19

Figure 8.9*b*.

liver and renal disease. During the interaction, in which CADU-
CEUS asked for additional data, the program first "recognized"
that liver disease was involved, created a list of diseases that could
account for the findings, and then undertook the resolution of the
renal findings. After eliminating several diseases on the basis of
further information supplied it, it asked the question, "What was
the result of a leptospira agglutination test?" Upon being informed that this specific test was positive, CADUCEUS made the
diagnosis of hepatic and renal leptospirosis. This program gives
the appearance of going through the data, creating hypotheses,
seeking further data, and then testing the hypotheses against the
data, in much the same way a physician seems to.

When the positive disease attributes used by CADUCEUS were

Terms entered into RECONSIDER

ascites, selectivity = 0.958
pedal edema, selectivity = 0.999
pitting, selectivity = 0.996
alcohol, selectivity = 0.971
hepatomegaly, selectivity = 0.929
chest pain, selectivity = 0.950
exertional dyspnea, selectivity = 0.983
orthopnea, selectivity = 0.986
neck veins, selectivity = 0.991
kussmaul, selectivity = 0.997
calcification, selectivity = 0.845

	10.604	—	maximum total score		562 diseases

1	6.688	pericarditis, constrictive	04
2	2.946	hemopericardium	04
3	2.933	heart, tamponade	04
4	2.927	myocarditis, active	04
5	2.891	pulmonary valve, stenosis	04
6	2.878	amyloidosis, primary, nonhereditary	00
7	2.878	heart, failure, congestive	04
8	2.873	tricuspid valve, stenosis	04
9	2.873	cor pulnonale	04-03
10	2.858	liver, cirrhosis, portal	06

PIP's diagnoses   FIT:

1. constrictive pericarditis   0.78
2. congestive heart failure   0.44

Figure 8.9c.

supplied to RECONSIDER, it processed them and generated a disease list beginning:

1. liver, cirrhosis, portal   score 11.141
2. liver, massive necrosis   9.300
3. leptospirosis   9.208

.
.
.

The inclusion of the correct diagnosis near the top of the computed disease list was considered a satisfactory performance even though in its present form RECONSIDER could not request further data in an attempt to assist in improving the differential. In generating this list, it considered approximately ten times as many candidate diseases as did CADUCEUS.

The more interesting question is, How could such a simple program as RECONSIDER do so well? Is there some magical power in the mere use of words which makes this possible? In a sense there is, but it is neither magical nor beyond our understanding. When physicians describe diseases, they use carefully chosen words in their descriptions. As they question and examine patients, the abnormalities they find are described with the use of these specific and particular terms. Physicians use such terms as *murmur, bruit, ronchi,* or *rales* rather than such general words as *sounds* or *noise,* and their choice of the descriptive terms to be used is an advance toward a diagnosis. Their perceptions of these clinical observables, created during a wholly prelinguistic phase, are formed and shaped so that these links between objects and words fall into place. RECONSIDER is, of course, an entirely non-AI program, and it makes no pretense of modeling any cognitive processes. Its performance, we would suggest, depends upon the human intelligence that was earlier invested by the CMIT authors in their disease descriptions, and then later by the clinicians in their descriptions of the clinical attributes they ascribed to their patients. The program itself does no more than estimate the similarity between a disease description and a patient description. It is probable, of course, that physicians do something like this during diagnosis.

From this conclusion a warning emerges. We hypothesize that RECONSIDER works as well as it does because physicians have a rich, expressive, and specific vocabulary to select from when they describe particular clinical objects. If this is true, it follows that any paraphrasing or truncating applied to these descriptions will result in the loss of information and a degrading of the quality of the description. Since the process of coding enables us to represent a class of objects with a smaller number of symbols, we clearly lose information by coding. We can reduce this loss by increasing the number of symbols used in codes, but if this is extended to the point where every clinical term had a unique code there would be little value in coding. Because of the specificity of medical terms, there are advantages in representing medical meanings by the direct use of medical terms. If we were able to process medical information by retaining the clinician's original descriptions (i.e., avoiding coding), we might hope to avoid the information degradation which this entails.

There are other applications of the property of term specificity. One is to the general information retrieval problem.[11] The vector representation of the word-object relationships found in CMIT can be used in selecting from a mixture of medical terms those terms used in describing diseases of particular body systems. In this way we can algorithmically generate vocabularies that are specific for particular disease categories (or for the literature of the corresponding medical subspecialties), as shown in figure 8.10. Such specialty vocabularies can then be employed as recognition vocabularies for the searching and recognition of unindexed medical text. If the text of an abstract or an article is compared word by word to a set of such recognition vocabularies (specific for different subjects), it should be possible to allocate the text to the subject

Title: Epidermolysis Bullosa Acquista
Id: Arch Derm103, 1-10, 1971

Epidermolysis bullosa acquista (EBA) is a rare, nonhereditary, blistering disease
     01   01   08
with clinical features similar to epidermolysis bullosa dystrophica. The clinical
                  01   01
features may often simulate porphyria cutanea tarda, pemphigus, or pemphigoid.
               00   01
Three new cases of EBA are discussed. The first patient had signs of a "lymphoma-like" disorder of lymph nodes. The other two patients had inflammatory disorders of the gastrointestinal tract. A review of all other reported cases of EBA shows a high incidence of associated systemic disease, amtloidosis, colitis,
                                       06
enteritis, multiple myeloma, and diabetes mellitus.
   06

Program assigned: Integumentary. Editor assigned: Dermatology.

Total hit vector — 1 5 0 0 0 0 2 0 1 0 0
Total hits — 9   Total words — 85

Figure 8.10. The output of a text classification program that processed the abstract shown. The program used recognition vocabularies specific for each disease category; the recognized words have the corresponding category number printed beneath them (see text).

A	MMij	Pij	Oo	Op	Pi	Oi	Pj	Oj	Wi-Wj
0.8954	8	.90	(8 ,	0)	.00	(14)	.00	(8)	kernig-brudzinski
0.8592	7	.89	(7 ,	0)	.03	(96)	.00	(7)	rales-rhonchi
0.8587	13	.87	(12 ,	0)	.01	(25)	.00	(13)	polyuria-polydipsia
0.8547	5	.86	(5 ,	0)	.00	(7)	.00	(5)	chvostek-trousseau
0.8195	5	.86	(5 ,	0)	.04	(122)	.00	(5)	convulsions-trousseau
0.8147	7	.89	(7 ,	0)	.07	(241)	.00	(7)	cough-rhonchi
0.8110	4	.83	(4 ,	1)	.02	(72)	.00	(4)	constipation-aches
0.8057	5	.86	(5 ,	0)	.05	(167)	.00	(5)	bleeding-hemartaroses
0.7988	3	.80	(3 ,	0)	.00	(3)	.00	(3)	egotism-greediness
0.7985	3	.80	(3 ,	0)	.00	(4)	.00	(3)	distrust-egotism
0.7985	3	.80	(3 ,	0)	.00	(4)	.00	(3)	distrust-greediness
0.7975	3	.80	(3 ,	0)	.00	(7)	.00	(3)	maladjustment-apathetic
0.7957	3	.80	(3 ,	0)	.00	(13)	.00	(3)	blisters-photosensitivity
0.7936	3	.80	(3 ,	0)	.01	(20)	.00	(3)	exophthalmos-apathetic
0.7887	3	.80	(3 ,	0)	.01	(36)	.00	(3)	apathy-apathetic
0.7877	3	.80	(3 ,	0)	.01	(39)	.00	(3)	stupor-apathetic
0.7825	3	.80	(3 ,	0)	.02	(56)	.00	(3)	delirium-apathetic
0.7740	3	.80	(3 ,	0)	.03	(84)	.00	(3)	hypertension-proteinuria
0.7736	4	.83	(4 ,	0)	.06	(194)	.00	(4)	malaise-afebrile
0.7733	3	.80	(3 ,	0)	.03	(86)	.00	(3)	murmur-corrigan
0.7700	3	.80	(3 ,	0)	.03	(97)	.00	(3)	coma-apathetic
0.7680	7	.78	(6 ,	0)	.01	(31)	.00	(7)	hemiplegia-monoplegia
0.7592	46	.83	(39 ,	0)	.07	(241)	.01	(46)	cough-wheezing

Figure 8.11. Most highly associated pairs of words used in the symptoms and signs parts of CMIT. The left-most column is the computed association coefficient for the pair of words shown on the right. The parenthesized numbers in the fourth column represent, respectively, the observed number of word co-occurrences (Oo) and the number of co-occurrences (Op) predicted on the basis of the two single term frequencies. (See text for more complete explanation.)

area it most closely resembles. In one experiment with recognition vocabularies of this kind, we simply counted "hits" between the texts of abstracts and a set of eleven such vocabularies, and used a uniform weighting scheme. Using a simple program, a series of abstracts taken from different medical specialty journals was correctly allocated to the subject matter field in two-thirds of the cases. It was interesting to find that when the classification assigned by the program differed from that of a human editor the algorithmic classification seemed, in many cases, at least as appropriate as the human classification. One abstract so classified is shown in figure 8.10. This particular abstract was taken from the *Archives of Dermatology,* but the program assigned the text to "gastroenterology" rather than to "dermatology." Inspection of the abstract will show this to be an appropriate assignment. A somewhat similar approach has been described by K. A. Hamill and A. Zamora [52] for the classification of journal articles (using only the titles) among the section headings used in *Chemical Abstracts.*

A question of some importance in the development of diagnostic programs (and in diagnosis, when made by humans) is that of the independence of disease attributes. A question we raised earlier asked whether the relations occurring among objects in the world tend to be reflected in the structure of our descriptions of these objects. Specifically, if the attributes of a particular disease are related through pathophysiological mechanisms, might we hope to be able to detect this by algorithmic means from an examination of the descriptions of diseases? The question is whether a patient's having a particular attribute will affect the likelihood of finding another one to be present. For example, if a patient is found to have "polyarthritis," is "fever" likely to be present by more than pure chance? Here the intuitive answer would seem to be yes, but only with the proviso that this likelihood may depend upon the presence or absence of other attributes as well.

If a patient complained of "nausea," we would expect episodes of "vomiting" to be associated with this. Nausea and vomiting go together. But "diplopia" and "pruritus" have no such natural connection. Underlying the pathophysiologic account of a particular disease there will be causal connections among attributes which, as with "nausea" and "vomiting," underlie their co-occurrence. If, however, we were to find in a patient clinical abnormalities that were not so easily related, say, "diplopia" and "pruritus," we would be inclined to postulate two different disease processes. Because of our commitment during diagnosis to the principle of parsimony, we might be tempted to choose one of these as being the significant finding and dismiss the other as a red herring.[12]

All physicians know (or quickly learn) the most common disease-attribute pairs, and the important clusters of symptoms and signs that tend to be found together. The discovery of other such pairs or clusters will increase as our knowledge of pathophysiology grows. But when we consider that there are several thousand disease attributes of importance (including symptoms, signs, and laboratory findings), the resulting millions of attribute pairs will *always* remain beyond the capacity of human memory.[13] Moreover, we may not know enough about the biology underlying certain disease attributes to be able to analyze the clinical problem causally. What we would like to know, then, is whether particular attribute pairs or clusters occur at rates substantially greater or rarer than would be predicted by chance alone. This information is not yet generally available, though it will be eventually, as large-scale clinical data bases come into common use.

Yet there is another approach which, if not as direct, would appear to offer promise. In the CMIT descriptions of diseases, the characteristic disease attributes listed were obtained in the first place from the direct clinical study of individual patients. Might we then, by using the descriptions of diseases, estimate the attribute co-occurrence frequencies, and assume that these will reflect, even approximately, the underlying connections among these attributes as found in clinical practice? In a pilot experiment, we took 1,000 low-entropy terms from the symptoms and signs list, and created a list of half a million word pairs. A program was then written to count the number of word co-occurrences when they co-occurred *anywhere* within a single disease description. An association measure was then defined and computed that compared the observed term co-occurrence rates with those expected from chance alone (computed from their known single-term frequencies).

When we computed these association coefficients for term pairs and sorted this list of half a million pairs in decreasing value of the association measure, we obtained the results shown in part in figures 8.11 and 8.12. The pairs at the top of the list have large positive-association measures. They occur together much more frequently than would be expected on the basis of chance alone. In fact, the term pairs shown are more tightly correlated than "nausea" and "vomiting," a standard example of a pair of closely related attributes.

From the manner in which we defined our measure, a word pair will have a high association value even if each word occurs singly fairly frequently, provided only that they co-occur at a rate substantially greater than expected. It may also be high when the words are uncommon and the number of observed co-occurrences is small provided, again, the number expected by chance is still less. As examples, the positively correlating pair "cough" and "wheezing" occurs *as single words* in 241 different diseases and 46 different diseases, respectively. On the basis of these single-term frequencies, we would expect to find three joint occurrences by chance alone, and yet we find that there are thirty-nine of them. For less common terms, such as *corrigan* and *austin-flint* (where the latter is treated as a single word), which occur singly in only three and two diseases, respectively, they are found to co-occur in two diseases, and thus have a high association value because of the near zero probability of this occurring by chance. Our hypothesis that term pairs such as these should have high co-occurrence rates because of underlying causal connections thus seems to be borne out.

Examining the list in figure 8.11 more carefully reveals other features. The co-occurrence "argyll-robertson" is in a sense an artifact, since this particular pair of words is semantically a single term.[14] Most surprising, perhaps, is that the pairs whose single terms are extremely rare (e.g., "agrammatism-paraphasia," in which the single terms occur only twice, but both times within the same description), may have high co-occurrence rates that make sense clinically. This appears surprising because our intuition becomes poor when we deal with very small probabilities (near zero). Given the small numbers of the observed co-occurrences of some of these term pairs, we might have supposed that some biologically unrelated word pairs would appear near the top of the list through chance alone. But this did not happen, and the likelihood of its occurring can be shown to be remote.

What, then, is the significance of word pairs that have large

A	MMij	Pij	Oo Op	Pi	Oi	Pj	Oj	Wi-Wj
−0.0872	55	.02	(0 , 5)	.10	(341)	.02	(55)	dyspnea-knee
−0.0872	65	.03	(1 , 7)	.12	(381)	.02	(65)	bone-atrial
−0.0867	64	.03	(1 , 7)	.12	(381)	.02	(64)	bone-urethral
−0.0867	97	.03	(2 , 11)	.12	(381)	.03	(97)	bone-sounds
−0.0867	31	.03	(0 , 3)	.12	(381)	.01	(31)	bone-perineum
−0.0867	31	.03	(0 , 3)	.12	(381)	.01	(31)	bone-ovary
−0.0866	53	.02	(0 , 5)	.10	(341)	.02	(53)	dyspnea-cystoscopy
−0.0866	53	.02	(2 , 5)	.10	(341)	.02	(53)	dyspnea-disk
−0.0860	53	.02	(0 , 5)	.10	(341)	.02	(53)	dyspnea-nystagmous
−0.0865	129	.03	(3 , 15)	.12	(381)	.04	(129)	bone-artery
−0.0863	52	.02	(0 , 5)	.10	(341)	.02	(52)	dyspnea-genitalia
−0.0861	95	.03	(2 , 11)	.12	(381)	.03	(95)	bone-ventricle
−0.0858	30	.03	(0 , 3)	.12	(381)	.04	(30)	bone-angiocardiography
−0.0858	62	.03	(1 , 7)	.12	(381)	.02	(62)	bone-conjunctiva
−0.0858	30	.03	(0 , 3)	.12	(381)	.01	(30)	bone-leads
−0.0858	30	.03	(0 , 3)	.12	(381)	.01	(30)	bone-exertional
−0.0855	50	.02	(0 , 5)	.10	(341)	.02	(50)	dyspnea-penis
−0.0855	50	.02	(0 , 5)	.10	(341)	.02	(50)	dyspnea-behavior
−0.0853	61	.03	(1 , 7)	.12	(381)	.02	(61)	bone-diaphragm
−0.0848	29	.03	(0 , 3)	.12	(381)	.01	(29)	bone-gallop
−0.0843	29	.03	(0 , 3)	.12	(381)	.01	(29)	bone-pupil
−0.0868	60	.03	(1 , 7)	.12	(381)	.02	(60)	bone-waves
−0.0848	29	.03	(0 , 3)	.12	(381)	.01	(29)	bone-gallbladder

Figure 8.12. Lowest associated pairs of words used in the symptoms and signs parts of CMIT. (See caption for fig. 8.11 for explanation.)

negative association values (fig. 8.12). Taking the single words in the pair at the very bottom, "bone-gallbladder," which have individual occurrence frequencies of 381 and 29, respectively, we would have expected three co-occurrences by chance and we found none. But there is no reason why we should find these words as a pair in the description of any single disease. There are simply no diseases that require the use of both of these words in describing them.

During the process of diagnosis we use information beyond that obtained from histories and physical examinations. Although the 1971 edition of CMIT which we used is now quite out of date with respect to clinical laboratory procedures, we were interested in extending the valuation of our underlying hypothesis by examining the association of term pairs taken from the laboratory part of CMIT. These term pairs were processed using the methods described, and the top and bottom of the term-pair list, in order of decreasing association measure, is shown in figures 8.13 and 8.14. The relatedness of the words in pairs on the first list, and the unrelatedness of those in the second will again be readily apparent to the physician reader. As a final experiment, word pairs were then formed by taking the first term from the symptoms and signs parts of CMIT, and the second term from the laboratory part. These associations are shown in figures 8.15 and 8.16, and the results are subject to the same comments as above.

When Bayes' Theorem[15] is employed in diagnostic programs, one of the simplifying assumptions commonly made is that disease attributes are independent of one another. In making this assumption, it is usually granted that this cannot be true. This assumption would be true only for word pairs having association values in the neighborhood of zero. If a patient exhibits two clinical attributes that are not independent (because of underlying causal relationships, whether they happen to be known or not), the observation of the second attribute does not add as much information (in the Hartley-Shannon sense) as it would in the absence of knowledge of the first. As an example (see fig. 8.11), if we knew that a patient had Kernig's sign, the further finding of Brudzinski's sign would not provide as much information as if the latter had been the only finding.

These semantic properties of medical words, which we assumed to reflect the connections between words and objects, and the fur-

A	MMij	Pij	Oo Op	Pi Oi	Pj Oj	Wi-Wj
0.9311	41	.98	(41, 1)	.05 (148)	.01 (41)	ecg-qrs
0.9110	20	.95	(20, 0)	.04 (141)	.01 (20)	csf-pleocytosis
0.9089	20	.95	(20, 0)	.05 (148)	.01 (20)	ecg-interval
0.9067	19	.95	(19, 0)	.05 (148)	.01 (19)	ecg-p-r
0.8995	12	.93	(12, 0)	.03 (94)	.00 (12)	marrow-erythroid
0.8988	16	.94	(16, 0)	.05 (148)	.01 (16)	ecg-inverted
0.8988	16	.94	(16, 0)	.05 (148)	.01 (16)	ecg-st
0.8972	37	.97	(37, 2)	.08 (251)	.01 (37)	ophthalmoscopy-disk
0.8800	9	.91	(9, 0)	.03 (94)	.00 (9)	marrow-normoblastic
0.8710	10	.92	(10, 0)	.05 (148)	.00 (10)	ecg-bundle-branch
0.8634	9	.91	(9, 0)	.05 (148)	.00 (9)	ecg-premature
0.8606	30	.91	(28, 1)	.05 (148)	.01 (30)	ecg-axis
0.8598	7	.89	(7, 0)	.03 (94)	.00 (7)	marrow-myelocytes
0.8563	49	.90	(45, 2)	.05 (148)	.02 (49)	ecg-t
0.8547	5	.86	(5, 0)	.00 (7)	.00 (5)	acth-17-hydroxycorticoid
0.8544	8	.90	(8, 0)	.05 (148)	.00 (8)	ecg-vl
0.8544	8	.90	(8, 0)	.05 (148)	.00 (8)	ecg-q-t
8.8513	5	.86	(5, 4)	.01 (18)	.00 (5)	pbi-radioiodine
0.8486	5	.86	(5, 0)	.01 (27)	.00 (5)	vital-o2
0.8480	13	.87	(12, 0)	.02 (60)	.00 (13)	time-tourniquet
0.8462	35	.89	(32, 1)	.05 (148)	.01 (35)	ecg-deviation
0.8461	5	.86	(5, 0)	.01 (35)	.00 (5)	capacity-o2
0.8459	6	.88	(6, 0)	.03 (94)	.00 (6)	marrow-hypercellular
0.8459	6	.88	(6, 0)	.03 (94)	.00 (6)	marrow-myeloblasts

Figure 8.13. Highest associated pairs of words, both taken from the laboratory parts of CMIT. (See caption for fig. 8.11 for explanation.)

A	MMij	Pij	Oo	Op	Pi	Oi	Pj	Oj	Wi-Wj
−0.0322	109	.05	(4 ,	8)	.08	(251)	.03	(109)	ophthalmoscopy-biopsy
−0.0318	20	.05	(0 ,	1)	.08	(251)	.01	(20)	ophthalmoscopy-iodine
−0.0318	20	.05	(0 ,	1)	.08	(251)	.01	(20)	ophthalmoscopy-flocculation
−0.0307	41	.05	(1 ,	3)	.08	(251)	.01	(41)	ophthalmoscopy-qrs
−0.0305	148	.05	(6 ,	11)	.08	(251)	.05	(148)	ophthalmoscopy-ecg
−0.0300	62	.02	(0 ,	2)	.05	(148)	.02	(62)	ecg-pyuria
−0.0296	19	.05	(0 ,	1)	.08	(251)	.01	(19)	ophthalmoscopy-p-r
−0.0292	13	.07	(0 ,	1)	.10	(312)	.00	(13)	wbc-cytology
−0.0288	60	.05	(2 ,	4)	.08	(251)	.02	(60)	ophthalmoscopy-time
−0.0272	18	.05	(0 ,	1)	.08	(251)	.01	(18)	ophthalmoscopy-pbi
−0.0272	18	.05	(0 ,	1)	.08	(251)	.01	(18)	ophthalmoscopy-amylase
−0.0262	58	.02	(0 ,	2)	.04	(141)	.02	(58)	csf-waves
−0.0262	27	.03	(0 ,	1)	.06	(197)	.01	(27)	anemia-vital
−0.0257	141	.03	(4 ,	8)	.06	(197)	.04	(141)	anemia-cst
−0.0249	26	.04	(0 ,	1)	.06	(197)	.01	(26)	anemia-laryngoscopy
−0.0248	94	.02	(1 ,	4)	.05	(148)	.03	(94)	ecg-marrow
−0.0247	141	.02	(2 ,	6)	.05	(148)	.04	(141)	ecg-csf
−0.0246	17	.05	(0 ,	1)	.08	(251)	.01	(17)	ophthalmoscopy-eosinophils
−0.0245	26	.07	(1 ,	2)	.10	(312)	.01	(26)	wbc-bronchoscopy
−0.0243	13	.07	(0 ,	1)	.09	(296)	.00	(13)	blood-proctoscopy
−0.0243	13	.07	(0 ,	1)	.09	(296)	.00	(13)	blood-crystals
−0.0227	53	.05	(2 ,	4)	.08	(251)	.02	(53)	ophthalmoscopy-thrombocytopenia
−0.0221	83	.02	(1 ,	3)	.05	(148)	.03	(83)	ecg-rbc
−0.0218	44	.02	(0 ,	1)	.04	(141)	.01	(44)	caf-p
−0.0218	94	.01	(0 ,	3)	.03	(104)	.03	(94)	culture-marrow
−0.0217	16	.06	(0 ,	1)	.08	(251)	.01	(16)	ophthalmoscopy-bsp

Figure 8.14. Low association end (bottom) of the same list from which figure 8.13 shows the top. (See caption of fig. 8.11 for explanation.)

A	MMij	Pij	Oo	Op	Pi	Oi	Pj	Oj	Wi-Wj
0.8727	7	.89	(7	, 0)	.02	(52)	.00	(7)	rash-weil-felix
0.8565	8	.90	(8	, 0)	.04	(141)	.00	(8)	csf-brudzinski
0.8544	26	.93	(25	, 2)	.07	(241)	.01	(26)	cough-bronchoscopy
0.8444	6	.88	(6	, 0)	.03	(99)	.00	(6)	pallor-hypercellular
0.8385	5	.86	(5	, 0)	.02	(68)	.00	(5)	time-hemarthroses
0.8315	14	.88	(13	, 0)	.04	(141)	.00	(14)	csf-kernig
0.8309	4	.83	(4	, 0)	.00	(7)	.00	(4)	xanthomas-betalipoproteins
0.8274	5	.86	(5	, 0)	.03	(96)	.00	(5)	rales-o2
0.8241	13	.87	(12	, 0)	.04	(138)	.00	(13)	jaundice-sgpt
0.8115	5	.86	(5	, 0)	.05	(148)	.00	(5)	ecg-heave
0.8027	10	.83	(9	, 0)	.03	(99)	.00	(10)	pallor-anisocytosis
0.8004	9	.82	(9	, 0)	.02	(57)	.00	(9)	hematuria-papanicolaou
0.7982	3	.80	(3	, 0)	.00	(5)	.00	(3)	radioiodine-apathetic
0.7978	4	.83	(4	, 0)	.04	(115)	.00	(4)	hepatomegaly-metamyelocytes
0.7975	3	.80	(3	, 0)	.00	(7)	.00	(3)	xanthomas-glycerides
0.7975	3	.80	(3	, 0)	.00	(7)	.00	(3)	xanthomas-phla
0.7957	3	.80	(3	, 0)	.00	(10)	.00	(3)	polydipsia-dehydration
0.7942	3	.80	(3	, 0)	.01	(18)	.00	(3)	pbi-apathetic
0.7938	4	.83	(4	, 0)	.04	(128)	.00	(4)	splenomegaly-metamyelocytes
0.7938	4	.83	(4	, 0)	.04	(128)	.00	(4)	splenomegaly-peroxidase
0.7931	29	.84	(25	, 1)	.05	(148)	.01	(4)	ecg-gallop
0.7920	3	.80	(3	, 0)	.01	(25)	.00	(3)	polyuria-dehydration
0.7911	3	.80	(3	, 0)	.01	(28)	.00	(3)	bmr-apathetic

Figure 8.15. Pairs of words having the highest association values, where the words may occur in any part of the CMIT disease description. (See caption of fig. 8.11 for explanation.)

A	MMij	Pij	Oo , Op	Pi	Oi	Pj	Oj	Wi-Wj
−0.0397	21	.04	(0 , 1)	.07	(241)	.01	(21)	cough-platelets
−0.0301	111	.01	(0 , 4)	.04	(126)	.03	(111)	paralysis-hematuria
−0.0297	44	.02	(0 , 2)	.05	(167)	.01	(44)	bleeding-p
−0.0287	57	.02	(0 , 2)	.05	(148)	.02	(57)	ecg-ataxia
−0.0287	42	.02	(0 , 2)	.05	(167)	.01	(42)	bleeding-wave
−0.0267	101	.09	(4 , 7)	.02	(251)	.03	(101)	ophthalmoscopy-frequency
−0.0265	69	.01	(0 , 2)	.04	(181)	.02	(69)	csf-dysuria
−0.0284	39	.05	(1 , 3)	.03	(251)	.01	(39)	ophthalmoscopy-amenorrhea
−0.0262	41	.02	(0 , 2)	.05	(167)	.01	(41)	bleeding-qrs
−0.0279	11	.08	(0 , 1)	.10	(341)	.03	(11)	dyspnea-rhinoscopy
−0.0272	36	.05	(0 , 3)	.03	(251)	.01	(39)	ophthalmoscopy-petechiae
−0.0252	101	.32	(1 , 4)	.05	(148)	.03	(101)	ecg-frequency
−0.0259	58	.32	(0 , 2)	.04	(138)	.32	(58)	jaundice-papilledena
−0.0259	37	.03	(0 , 1)	.09	(167)	.01	(37)	bleeding-calcium
−0.0258	37	.03	(0 , 1)	.09	(167)	.01	(37)	bleeding-disk
−0.0252	47	.02	(0 , 2)	.05	(148)	.01	(47)	ecg-blindness
−0.0251	62	.03	(1 , 3)	.03	(183)	.02	(82)	cyanosis-pyuria
−0.0246	35	.05	(1 , 2)	.03	(251)	.01	(36)	ophthalmoscopy-anemia
−0.0246	69	.01	(0 , 2)	.04	(129)	.32	(68)	paralysis-alkaline
−0.0244	39	.03	(0 , 1)	.05	(167)	.31	(39)	bleeding-deviation
−0.0244	35	.03	(0 , 1)	.09	(167)	.01	(35)	bleeding-capacity
−0.0242	66	.01	(0 , 2)	.04	(128)	.02	(55)	paralysis-phosphatase

Figure 8.16. Low association end (bottom) of the same list from which figure 8.15 shows the top. (See caption of fig. 8.11 for explanation.)

ther connections among the objects, seem to be experimentally measurable. These are the very properties we count upon daily when we try to say just the right thing without saying either too much or too little, and as we attempt to avoid being overly general while at the same time being no more specific than is warranted. These features are essential in the process of reference, the process that we have considered with respect to the mappings we visualize between the world and our descriptions of it. Since the communication and processing of medical information is so influenced by this matter of description, we will consider some of the difficulties of creating descriptions and, in particular, with creating descriptions that we can use with a computer.

9

The Representation of
Medical Information

9.1 The Medical Record Problem and Medical Information Systems

Until relatively recent times, the recording of medical information (when this occurred at all) was carried out informally and as a matter of interest primarily to the physician. Such informal and personal records have served as the basis for clinical reports and for the teaching of medicine during the first two millennia of its history. With the advent of aseptic surgery and anesthesia, which drew surgery into the hospital, and of clinical pathology and radiology, which did much the same for internal medicine, three new features of medical communication emerged.

The increasing number of hospitals and polyclinics built during the latter half of the nineteenth century and the concurrent increase in medical knowledge made medical specialization not only feasible but essential. As large numbers of patients and physicians were brought together in these institutions, the provision of specialized clinical services and the use of specialist consultants became increasingly convenient. The patient-care process then began its evolution toward the referral and consultant system and toward the group or team processes we have today. The eighteenth-century physician, who may have performed as apothecary as well, began to evolve into the present-day medical manager. The treatment of the hospitalized patient became increasingly shared by the attending physician with consultants (clinical specialists and sub-specialists, radiologists, pathologists), nurses and, most recently, a variety of specialized therapists. This continuing division of labor has brought with it the need for increasingly formal means of communication among the participants in the medical-care process, and the hospital chart has evolved to fill this crucial integrative and communicative role.

The modern hospital, by bringing physicians into closer professional contact with one another, produced other results. Physicians were now working together and observing each others' performances at closer range than before, and this led gradually to the voluntary adoption of professional standards, first in the hospital and then, later, in the community. The medical record, which earlier served as the private diary of the attending physician and later as a "bulletin board" for the intercommunication of medical professionals, has now become an institutionalized and semipublic document. It is presently used by both the medical and hospital staffs for an increasing number of review and audit purposes, which takes it far beyond its primary role in patient care. In order to facilitate these processes, professional and hospital organizations have developed uniform standards of medical record-keeping, which they attempt to enforce.

A third use for medical records is found in the pursuit of clinical research. Although the physician's descriptions of disease courses and outcomes have served this purpose since they were introduced by Hippocrates, the accumulated clinical descriptions in medical record libraries have increasingly become a resource for researchers. Each of these reasons for keeping medical records, however imperfect the means, continues to increase in importance. As a result of this increasing activity, the competition among users for access to a particular medical record or to a single physical document has resulted in growing frustration.

What has not increased to a corresponding degree has been our effectiveness in creating, maintaining, and retrieving medical records, and in conveniently communicating medical data. It has now been some twenty years since the first significant steps were taken to apply computer and communication technology to this problem by developing what is now called a *Hospital Information System* (HIS) or, more generally, a *Medical Information System* (MIS). Such systems have been defined by Lindberg: "A medical information system is a set of formal arrangements by which facts concerning the health or health care of individual patients are stored and processed in computers'' [70]. As recent reviews of these systems have emphasized, they may take on myriad forms [47, 59]. Such a system need only carry out some single isolatable function, and it could be spoken of as constituting a module or subsystem of some larger actual or potential system. These elementary systems may then be further aggregated into larger systems serving more comprehensive purposes. Technically this may be accomplished by the networking of previously freestanding or otherwise autonomous systems, and this process of modular evolution, later followed by aggregation, is one of the two principal methods that have been proposed for the development of comprehensive medical information systems [7, 14].

An alternative approach has been to begin with the design of the large or more comprehensive system at the start, and to develop it all at once. Until fairly recently, the latter method has been the one most widely employed. The reason for this has been that the size and cost of a large mainframe computer (the only kind available in the 1960s) required that it support a substantial single computing load in order to justify the large investment. With the advent of minicomputers in the early 1970s and more recently of microcomputers, which have produced drastic decreases in computing costs, the construction of monolithic systems is now declining. Although there is a lower limit to the size or complexity of such systems, there is in principle no upper limit. Yet the most comprehensive of present systems perform only a fraction of the information processing tasks requiring attention within hospitals, and they fall far short of the ambitions expressed twenty years ago. The complete computerization of the hospital record remains to be accomplished, and Lindberg has identified a score of the specific information processes he regards as being impossible of computerization at the present time.

The development of MISs has been an expensive and frustrating undertaking, characterized by a hesitant and uncertain progress for two decades. The lack of progress at the rate originally hoped for is now well recognized, as Lindberg points out:

> M.I.S.'s based on computers have a potentially major contribution
> to make to health services research. Existing systems should be

viewed as partial examples of the ultimate potential. . . . The explanation of why this technology has not diffused smoothly into health care systems is complicated. [70]

Although the explanation cited by Lindberg may be complicated, one cause stands out clearly. While MIS projects promise to serve the interests of a mixed constituency, including hospital administrators, nurses, health-service researchers, government regulatory agencies, and clinical investigators, they have offered very little to the physician. Although they affect physicians differently, their adoption has been looked upon as more intrusive than helpful, at least until the past year or so. If these systems had offered physicians information support services that were truly useful, or if they had enabled them to perform their duties more effectively, this history might have been otherwise. But for a variety of conceptual and technical reasons, the functions the earlier MISs performed best were those which concerned physicians least. Lindberg's appraisal of present medical information systems after two decades of development reflects the widely held opinion that much remains to be accomplished, and his list of "infeasible but potentially useful tasks" that remain to be computerized stands as an agenda for future research and development.

The formal evaluation of MISs has proceeded continuously throughout the period of development of these systems, since the sponsors of these expensive projects have naturally had a keen interest in determining what they were receiving for their money. In addition to the methodological difficulties enumerated by Lindberg, G. A. Giebink and L. L. Hurst surveyed twenty-eight medical computer projects, principally record-keeping systems, and identified a total of sixteen specific technical problems. [47] Ronald Henley and Gio Wiederhold, in a study of automated ambulatory record systems, cited additional technical and management obstacles. [59] Despite these efforts to draw attention to the need for understanding the nature of these unsolved technical problems, there has been a persistent tendency to ignore them.

The cost-benefit analyses of complex computer-based information systems are particularly sensitive to the definitions employed for "cost" and for "benefit." For an MIS, one might hope to compare the development, capital, and operating costs of the system with the direct savings in labor and other costs realized by the system over its projected lifetime. On the cost side, there are a number of items that may be difficult to evaluate; for example, the uncompensated time and effort of the medical and hospital staffs during planning and implementation. Meaningful measures of savings are likewise difficult to determine, because the replaced human labor (if any) almost always contributed functions beyond those which are provided by the newly installed computer system. A ward clerk at a nursing station, though primarily employed to transcribe orders, file clinical documents, and maintain certain records (all of which an information system might do), will also answer telephone calls from patients' relatives, direct visitors to the patients' rooms, call the housekeeping department if a tray of food is spilled on the floor, and perform other extemporaneous tasks which no information system can do. The gulf between the high-level description of human tasks (such as an employee's job description) and the formal descriptions (flowcharts, computer programs) and abstractions that can be carried down to low levels, is a formidable one to bridge. To repeat Churchman's observation, it is no easy matter for a computer to replace a clerk.

If what is to count as a benefit of some computer system is broadened to include reduced communication error rates, increased retrievability of data, improved readability of laboratory or other reports and, perhaps most important, simple convenience, then the measurement of benefit becomes very uncertain. How does one go about computing the dollar value to the hospital of avoiding a mistranscribed drug order or a misidentified patient? In the absence of such measuring devices, indirect measurements such as overall costs must be used, together with still higher-level (and less certain) outcome measurements. In evaluating the usefulness of systems employed in high-level processes like medical care, which are subject to the vagaries of human behavior, it is not surprising that evaluations frequently seem unconvincing. It is difficult to judge the utility of MISs based on such analyses, and it may be more profitable to examine individual instances of success and failure. In the long run, it seems likely that the most useful test will be that of the marketplace itself.

Most of the problems singled out by Lindberg as having retarded the development of useful MISs, are technological (including conceptual and procedural). Most of these center about:

1. Suitable methods for representing the meanings of medical terms, or of natural language statements.
2. Improved means of man-machine communication.

From an information point of view, these are not unrelated; one deals with the representation of meaning, the other with its transmission across an interface. One way of accomplishing the former has been to encode the data of interest using a symbol system in which a specific symbol refers to a single thing, and this thing is represented by only a single symbol. Thus, persons, places, and things, many of which are ambiguously named, must be assigned unique symbols or codes. "John Jones" may be represented by 96-42-37, "penicillin-G" by 0483, and "pneumococcal-pneumonia" by 241. This approach requires that these equivalences be defined to the system and to users of the system. It also requires a great deal of human labor to perform the tedious and expensive translation from one rich but fuzzy representation (natural language) to another (the arbitrary codes chosen).

Only when all of the data have been so represented can processing proceed by use of algorithms, which are explicitly represented in the programs. These two features (precise symbol allocation, and algorithmic processing) taken together are what is meant by "computing." In contrast with the use of symbols in most bookkeeping and commercial applications in which the same symbols are used in both manual and computer systems, the representation of clinical information has a number of limitations. The available symbols (codes) rarely match the clinical data precisely, so that the user will frequently have to "force" the data into categories that may not be appropriate. Some important medical information may not be codable at all, which means it cannot be entered into an information system in a processible form. At present, much of the information obtained by history-taking or from the physical examination of the patient continues to be of this kind.

Consider the process of coding medical data from an information viewpoint. One consequence is the obvious one that coding introduces an additional level of abstraction. Every medical fact to be coded is itself an abstraction of some situation or of a more complex and richer description. The medical record is an abstraction to begin with, and all physicians are familiar with the difficulty of attempting to reconstruct the details of past events from this source alone. As difficult as this is, the use of natural language in this document provides a richer source of information than that resulting from further abstraction and coding. There are only a finite number of codes into which a near infinite number of meanings must be mapped. The result is that, when different things all map into the same code representation, it results in the irreversible loss of information. One cannot thereafter work backward and decide which of the meanings the code was used for, at least without additional information, which is external to the code itself. Conventional diagnostic coding does permit us, at some later time, to count mechanically the number of appendectomies performed in a hospital during a given period (though we may not be able to learn how many were necessary). And if, at that time, other data had been accurately recorded as well, we might be able to go on and learn who performed the appendectomies, and compute the average lengths of stay of patients and their complication rates. But much of the information in a chart or in an operation report cannot be readily coded, and so cannot be stored in machine-processible form. Every step in abstraction, by throwing away bits of the truth and reducing the information content of the description, limits the uses that may be made of the record at some future time. When we classify (which is what coding is) an object of interest, we are always at risk of distorting it. It would be a mistake to regard coded data, just because they appear so sharp and definite, as having the same information content as the original descriptions from which they were encoded. These difficulties are very much reduced when we have lower-level descriptions to begin with, which is why laboratory data are more effectively represented and stored, and why clinical laboratory information systems are so effective. However, the coding process is a costly one and, while it is presently necessary if computer systems are to be used at all for the processing of clinical data, the cost sets a limit to the use of processed clinical data. Entering high-level clinical information into computer systems is the most unsatisfactory step of all. While physicians have developed efficient and convenient means of communicating clinical facts to other physicians, scant progress has been made in improving the means for "communicating" these directly to computers. Because of the importance of the representation process and the disadvantages of present coding methods, major portions of the hospital record are not readily stored in computer-processible form, and it is this that stands in the way of a completely computerized medical record.

Some of the limitations of computer-based history-taking programs were considered in chapter 7. However, when histories are taken by physicians and expressed in natural language, there is *no* general method available for representing this information in processible form. Attempts to decompose a medical history or to summarize it synoptically with a problem list, which might be more easily codable, have been carried out, but these methods have not proven generally acceptable. The results of the physical examination, progress notes, and nursing notes are also not readily stored in processible form. The difficulty with all of these natural-language reports and observations is that they deal with the patient at too high a descriptive level. Symptoms and signs are high-level matters, and comments about a patient's mood or general condition are at even higher levels.

There are other kinds of clinical data, those which involve lower descriptive levels, and they are more easily represented with symbols. It was with these kinds of data that computers were first used in medicine, and where they have been most successful. The processing of physiological signals (patient monitoring, processing of ECGs) and of signals from analytical instruments (clinical chemistry) have been carried out with increasing effectiveness for two decades now. Since these are low-level patient attributes to begin with, the need for further abstraction does not arise. In addition, many of these attributes are obtained in numerical form initially, and are thus suitable for processing at once. One does not need to code low-level attributes of this sort, and those portions of the medical record which can be so expressed (which are, in a sense, self-coding), have been readily computerized. But as we have already noted, too, the use of low-level attributes *alone* is not a satisfactory way of describing high-level affairs. Only a limited number of diseases can be diagnosed from low-level attributes alone (e.g., from blood chemistries or blood counts), although these measurements may be crucial in following the course of many diseases.

When we have higher-level attributes like "pain," we may need to distinguish among "colicky," "cramping," "stabbing," "dull," and "sharp" pains, between "continuous" and "episodic" pain, and between "localized" and "radiating" pain. This is readily done using natural language, but even though these linguistic descriptions can be *stored* in computers, little further can be done with them at present. Some of the concepts discussed in chapter 8 with respect to the processing of words may provide help with this problem as future systems are developed.

9.2 The Formalization Gap

When we wish to computerize information processes in a particular application area, the first step is usually to carry out what is called a *systems analysis*. This procedure has two goals: the process in question must first be identified and isolated, and its boundaries fixed. Other processes with which the given one is directly coupled must be carefully detached, and all the connections that are severed must be clearly identified and labeled. When this isolation has been achieved, the target process or activity itself must be made completely explicit. The elements or subsystems of which it may be composed must be reduced to primitive form. When this has been done, it is a common practice to represent the results of these two steps in the form of a flow diagram or chart. Around the edges of this there will be lines representing the paths of information flow, which terminate abruptly. These are the connections which the process has with the rest of the world; they are the inputs and outputs representing the links with human operators or with other machines. Interior to these are the networks of interconnected boxes of various shapes representing the primitive information processes that connect the inputs and outputs.

The attempt to identify and isolate the obvious communication paths in hospitals may run into complex issues. Although it is easy enough to define the "official" channel for reporting the results of radiological examinations, there are parallel and "unofficial" channels as well. The most obvious of these is used when the attending physician, unwilling to wait for the official report, simply telephones the radiologist in the film viewing room. Or he may go there himself to get a "wet reading." Or, again, he may by chance meet the radiologist in the corridor shortly after the films were read, and be given the results informally. All except the first are "unofficial" channels, and one can think of many others that act in parallel with the official one. Several of these may provide a shorter response time, and others may provide an opportunity for asking additional questions. If a new official system (perhaps a computer-supported one) were to be designed and installed which proposed to reduce by half the previous response time, it is possible that the effect of such an improvement would pass unnoticed if these unofficial and parallel systems were heavily used. The actual flow of information in complex environments may be difficult to determine, the patterns of use of parallel or inapparent channels may be continually changing, and the construction and use of oversimplified models may do a great disservice.

There is always this conceptual gap between the real processes of medicine, between what actually goes on and the descriptions of them which we may hope to store or process. We can speak of this as a gap in formalization. This gap may be extremely wide in the case of the high-level processes and objects of medicine, but it narrows down in the case of the low-level ones. A serum potassium of 3.5 meq is a formal matter, but an irregular pulse is not, unless much more is said. It is the spanning of this formalization gap that is the task of representation, and the width of the gap is the measure of its difficulty.

It might be supposed that the conversion of high-level tasks into lower-level instructions is the job of programming languages. This seems to be only partially the case. The actual control of the computer hardware is exercised by a relatively small set of symbol strings or commands known as machine instructions. These are arbitrarily chosen by the machine designer to carry out the primitive operations of setting switches, opening or closing gates, and the like, in order to perform the primitive logic actions which, taken together, constitute the program. A computer can only respond to these primitive instructions, or machine code. The earliest users of computers wrote their programs directly in this machine code. It quickly became apparent that the process could be made much easier if combinations of frequently used processes could be invoked with the use of more comprehensive commands (higher-level instructions) such as "take the square root of x," and thus not require the programmer to indicate in detail all the individual additions, multiplications, and divisions (and their sequencing) that this operation entailed. So-called high-level languages were then developed that permitted the programmer to invoke still more complex processes and procedures with the use of single commands.

Because the computer hardware itself can only execute programs in machine code, it was necessary to develop still other kinds of programs, known as compilers, in order to process high-level languages. Compilers could accept a program written in a high-level language and convert it into an equivalent program expressed in machine code. Another means of accomplishing the same end, in the case of interactive systems is the use of interpreters. In more recent years, programming languages of greater expressivity and convenience have been developed, and some of these may be regarded as languages at a still higher level. The question is, can this "upward" evolution of programming languages be regarded as closing the formalization gap between programming languages and natural language? The answer, I believe, must be no. This evolution is simply headed in a different direction. High-level programming languages are no less formal than low-level machine languages.

Proposals have been made to develop methods for "automatic programming" in which an executable program could be automatically produced from a nonprocedural specification of the task to be performed. That is, instead of specifying the procedures to be used in attaining a desired goal, the goal itself would be formally specified. This approach has been carried out in certain instances with some success. AI programs for problem solving, such as MACSYMA,[1] have much of the desired flavor. In one sense, even these have not reduced the degree of formalization required since, instead of formalizing procedures, it becomes necessary to formalize tasks or goals. But the gap that needs closing is that between the informal and casual way in which humans carry out most of their everyday tasks, and the formal descriptions of these tasks or procedures which are necessary if a programmer is to have something with which to begin. Who is to fill this "formalization gap," then, as we attempt to build useful information systems in medicine?

Filling this gap has usually been done by systems analysts; by individuals familiar enough with the programmers' requirements to be able to create a formal description of a task and having at the same time enough understanding of a user's problem to make the final results fit the user's needs. The critical step in this formalization lies in the creation of appropriate abstractions, and this requires more than a casual acquaintance with the subject matter. In medicine, the professionals (physicians, nurses, pharmacists) are generally unaccustomed either by training or experience to create such abstractions in the form required by the programmer. It has been predicted that programmers will increasingly differentiate into one of two types: system programmers familiar with the inner workings of computers, their operating systems, and the software they support, and application programmers who will increasingly (and necessarily) become more expert in specific subject matter fields [133]. They properly emphasize the need for appropriate educational and training opportunities as a source of such skilled individuals, who will have a decreasing need for familiarity with the broad range of computer science, but a greatly increased need for specialty knowledge.[2]

This discontinuity in formalization between a manual (human) medical information process and the machine code necessary to accomplish comparable ends begins at a very high descriptive level and it is not itself a concern of computer science. If this concern is to be given a name at all, it must be regarded as concerning medical applications, and it is increasingly being referred to as "medical information science" in the United States, and as "medical informatics" in Europe. It will be the task of this new discipline to better understand and define the medical information processes we have considered here, in order that appropriate activities will be chosen for computerization, and to improve the man-machine system.

offer must more than offset the cost of learning how to use them. Because of this, the feasibility of introducing computer systems into the medical environment has been a subject of speculation since the earliest MISs were proposed. A number of assumptions were made at that time, and some have since become a part of the conventional wisdom. One was the assumption that physicians would not use a computer terminal with a conventional keyboard.[2] As a result of this, several current MISs which have been designed in the expectation that physicians would use the system themselves employ cathode ray tube (CRT) terminals operating with selection or "menu" lists, from which the desired functions can be individually indicated by means of a light pen (a small, penlike device which the physician need only point at a particular item on a menu to indicate the choice to the computer).

In the hospital with the longest continuous experience with such a system,[3] it has been reported that although some 60 percent of the staff physicians prefer the MISs to the previous manual procedures, the remainder do not. Although it requires more time to enter a set of orders directly into the MIS, the system, in return, offers the physician more rapid access to the laboratory and other diagnostic test results that are filed in the system. In exchange for a physician's willingness to learn how to use such a system, advantage is gained in being able to review parts of a patient's chart directly on the screen, and the ability to do this from remote locations. If an MIS could be accessed directly from a physician's office or home (via a dial-up telephone connection), it would offer physicians an added incentive to use these systems directly.

The convenience with which information systems are used depends significantly upon the skill with which the human engineering has been carried out. These efforts are necessarily constrained by the hardware and software available, and by the operating environment. If, for example, high-speed communication lines are available, the screen of a CRT terminal may be filled with text or tabular material retrieved from the computer in a second or less. With the low-speed lines most commonly available through the use of acoustic couplers and telephone lines, retrieval may require half a minute or so. If several large displays must be examined in sequence before some single option can be exercised, this delay first becomes annoying and then intolerable. Greater convenience can be obtained here but only by providing higher-speed communications.

To date there has been relatively little standardization in the procedures employed by different application systems, but with acceptance of these systems in the marketplace, standardization can be expected to grow. CRT terminals are becoming more alike in arrangement and in function and, as this continues, their acceptance by physicians will increase (as was the case with telephones and automobiles). Knowledge of the proper use of computers will be acquired by increasing numbers of people, and they will become regarded as familiar objects rather than as strange ones. The standardization of the procedures and protocols required for interacting with computers lags behind the physical makeup of terminals. This is probably because the design of these systems is still in ferment; alternative techniques are in competition, and the best choices are not yet clear.

The use of any powered device requires, at least in a metaphoric sense, that the user be capable of "communicating" with it. That is, a user must be able to command it to start and stop, to take this action and not some other and, in short, to have it perform in a desired way. For simple machines, which offer a user but few options, this "communication" is readily accomplished. Our very simplest powered devices need only on-off switches. More complex machines require further instructions, which may be effected by setting additional controls to particular values. The more complex the performance of a machine, the more numerous the required instructions become. In the domain of symbol manipulation—the generic process that computers can perform—the performance of complex problems would seem to have no upper limit. Any precisely definable symbol-manipulating process can be specified in a computer program. But this rich potential is available only to the programmer; once the program is in place, the previously general-purpose machine has been converted into a particular special-purpose one, and the actual user will perceive it as such.

Unlike many other special-purpose machines, the particular ends for which a computer system has been constructed are not readily apparent from the outside or by a casual inspection. They can only be determined from an examination of the program itself (which is its own best description), or from a user's manual. Even then, a computer system can only be understood by actually using it. It is here that the problems of the man-machine interface begin. Before using any machine, one needs to have a clear understanding of exactly what it is that the system is capable of doing. If the system is one of any significant subtlety, the task of describing its capabilities to the nonexpert is a far from simple one.

When a user concludes that a computer system appears able to do what is wanted, a detailed set of user instructions or directions must be available. These will begin with directions for "logging on" (and "off") the system, and authenticating that the user is an authorized user. This is commonly ensured by the use of assigned account numbers and passwords, although in a few early hospital systems it was done by issuing special keys or coded plastic cards to users. If the information system contains patient data, or if for whatever reason privacy is important, there may be several levels of access provided, which are appropriate for different kinds of users. There will also be different levels of access in order to protect the security and integrity of the system itself. Although access to a data base may be provided to many individuals, only certain personnel will be authorized to enter new data into the data base or to update existing records. Still fewer personnel will be afforded access to the programs themselves.

Once access to the system has been accomplished, there may be a number of different programs available, and the choice of which one a user desires must then be indicated. The designers of information systems generally arrange these matters so that within a particular system there is some uniformity and consistency among the procedures and protocols required to do these things. Designers will go to considerable lengths to make their system convenient or "user friendly." Yet these matters are relative, and a procedure that might appear logical or even intuitive to a programmer might be confusing and complex to someone having little experience with computers or computer languages.

One type of computer-based resource that seems certain to prove of widespread interest to physicians is the clinical data base. Such a data base will provide a particularly valuable collection of information, which at present can be accumulated only at considerable effort. Although it is difficult to foresee how the human engineering of such systems will proceed over the next decade, the kinds of problems that users will face can be predicted. In order to illustrate the different degrees of formalization involved in the use of clinical data base systems, we will consider some specific examples. In our Melanoma Clinic, a question that one physician might ask of another is:

1. "How many patients do you think we have seen in the Clinic who have initially presented with level-2 primaries and have gone on to die of their disease?"

This question is phrased here in the casual form in which such questions come to mind. The natural-language capability of the experimental data base system described previously (chap. 8) could provide an answer to this question if it were phrased only slightly less informally. At the present time it would have trouble with such words as *think, presented,* and *gone on to.* But let us paraphrase the question:

2. "How many patients with level-2 melanoma have died?"

This less complex question would promptly provide us with the desired answer. By transforming (1) into (2), we have made it possible for the natural-language program known as MEDINQUIRY to "understand" the inquiry, and to provide the answer. As with all computer programs, the quickest way for a user to become familiar with the capabilities and limitations of MEDINQUIRY is by using it. After a few minutes of introductory instruction, a completely inexperienced user is able to acquire a working knowledge of the system's capabilities. After a further hour or two of practice, a user is able to phrase inquiries quickly, knowing that they will be efficiently processed. The learning process required of a user of this program is informal and unstructured. It might be compared with the early exploratory phases of a conversation with a stranger using a foreign language in which we were only partially fluent. After exchanging a few remarks, we would have learned enough about our shared language capability to be able to phrase questions in such a way that they could be answered. The important point is that in both instances this familiarization occurs *informally.* This approach seems more convenient and natural than the alternative and formal one of being presented with lists of words that a computer will accept, and of the syntax that must be employed in using them. Learning by doing is a natural and effective process, and computer-based systems and programs that provide these kinds of introductions to their use will be particularly attractive.

In order to process inquiry (2) successfully, MEDINQUIRY requires the use of a large computer. If the entire machine is available for this sole use, the response time for an inquiry such as the one above is a few seconds, but if the computer is simultaneously serving other users, a response may require a minute or more. In order to make the retrieval process easy for the user, the system itself must do a great deal more work.

We have also been using a different, though similar, clinical data base in our Melanoma Clinic with much the same kinds of patient data in it, which utilizes the data-base management program INGRES [122], and which employs the retrieval language QUEL. Answering such questions as (2), above, using this data base is a much more structured undertaking than is the case when using MEDINQUIRY, since a formal retrieval language is required. To do this we must rephrase inquiry (2) in the formal language, QUEL, and obtain;

3. range of p is ptdata
   retrieve (deaths = count [p.ucnum where p.cstage = ''4a'' and p.lev = 2])

This inquiry would be meaningless to an unfamiliar user. However, the retrieval language is quickly learned, and someone with virtually no previous computer experience can learn how to use this system after a brief period of instruction and practice. The first line of (3) is a canonical form that informs the system of the data to be used. The second line simply indicates that what is wanted is the number of patient deaths, which is done by counting the number of medical record numbers assigned to patients with level-2 tumors, and whose current clinical stage is ''dead of melanoma.'' Once this modest investment in time and effort had been made a user would be capable of formulating other inquiries of comparable complexity. If the searching of the data base were to become a great deal more complex than this, or if particular kinds of output tables were desired, some further familiarization with the system would be necessary. The principal difference between queries (2) and (3) is that the programs supporting the latter type of inquiry can be run on a minicomputer or a microprocessor. These latter types of data-base management systems require more effort on the part of the user, but is then repaid by being able to employ less expensive hardware.

While (3) may appear mysterious to the uninitiated, the power offered by modern data-base management systems and their languages, like QUEL or its equivalents, is vastly superior to the earlier procedure of simply storing clinical data as it was organized in patient files. In order to obtain answers to questions like (1), (2), and (3) with conventional (flat-file) record-storage systems, it would be necessary to write (in an appropriate programming language) a retrieval program for each inquiry. If a large number of different clinical attributes were involved, it could take years and require the services of a full-time programmer in order to explore its contents completely. With the investment of a modest amount of time in learning how to use these more powerful systems, one clinical investigator alone could accomplish this in a matter of days if so inclined. And if access to a system having a natural-language capability were available, the required learning period would become insignificant.

As inquiry systems like these become easier to use and more widely available, one caution might seem to be in order. There is a risk inherent in these systems, which arises from the psychological power of the printed word, the mystique of the computer, and from the difficulty in tracing the connections between inquiries and answers. If the MEDINQUIRY system had printed out the answer "4" in response to inquiry (1), I would have accepted that, but if it had answered "40" I would not have. This is because I have a fairly detailed knowledge of the data stored in the system from having personally seen most of the patients from whom the data were obtained. I am also familiar with the ways in which the patient attributes were defined in the system, and how the retrieval is being carried out. In short, I would be able to interpret the results with more understanding than would someone unfamiliar with the system and the subject matter. If, however, I were performing retrievals with Fries's rheumatology system, I would be far less likely to spot a spurious result than would a rheumatologist. As information systems such as these, including diagnostic programs, become more widely employed by users who may be unfamiliar with the detailed contents and the conventions used, there is a danger that the results may be accorded a credibility which they do not deserve. Unfamiliarity becomes particularly risky when the output is merely a number or a name, and Shortliffe [115] has properly emphasized the need for such programs to be able to disclose in detail the means by which they arrive at "recommendations" or "diagnoses." Our natural tendency to accept a printed answer ("There it is in black and white!") could seriously undermine the credibility of computer aids in medicine unless special efforts were taken to ensure that their operation is transparent to the user. Fortunately, medicine has been faced with similar problems before, such as in the interpretation of laboratory test results, ECGs, or X-ray studies, and physicians are properly skeptical about answers that somehow do not seem to fit a situation.

In the effort to make computer systems easier to use, it is common practice to have the systems indicate when a user has made some mistake, by sending back "error messages." These can be very helpful to both casual users and fully trained system operators, especially when the messages are specific. But they must be understandable to the casual user, who is most in need of them. There have been proposals for using the methods of AI to make the man-machine interaction a smoother one. Natural language "front ends," spelling correctors, and the use of user-tolerant "default" procedures, all facilitate the more effective use of these systems.

10.2 Men and Machines in Information Processing

There are many aspects of this relationship between humans and their machines. At least two are of concern when we propose to automate information processes in medicine. One is the fact that before we can turn some task over to a machine, we must have first acquiesced in the replacement of an informal process by a formal one. This decision is more often made implicitly than explicitly, and in the case of unsuccessful projects it is a common reason for failure. One pays a price in accepting formalization, and the hope is that it will be less than the gains to be obtained. The price exacted may be in convenience, in being required to learn a new procedure, in functional rigidity, and almost always in a loss of information. Once a particular formalization has been agreed to, however, its incorporation into a machine process is usually straightforward if the formalization chosen is an appropriate one.

In agreeing to the formalization of some human task it must be remembered that it is no more than an abstraction of some real process or action, and that it will therefore always be incomplete. Automatic traffic signals always do less than traffic policemen do, and computerized billing systems do less than clerks. When, as in both of these cases, the machines do enough of the job to be useful, we can proceed to make the most of them.

A second point is that this incompleteness is a characteristic feature of all tools. Although a tool may do one or even several things better (i.e., cheaper, faster) than we can with our bare hands or unaided minds, no tool is expected to do everything that people do. In the extreme case of a hypothetical robot that could do "everything" that a human could, there would be no way of distinguishing the robot from the human. We would do well to regard robots that do less than this, and that exhibit the limitations characteristic of machines, as machines.

When we use machines to do some of the things (usually better) that we would otherwise do with our hands alone, we never bother to qualify these things with terms like *manual.* Although a bulldozer may accomplish the work of a score of manual laborers, we are not inclined to say that it is doing some manual task. When we employ a computer to do one or more of the many things for which we would ordinarily use our minds, there seems to be a compulsion to say that the computer is doing some "mental" thing, perhaps that it is "thinking," or even that it is displaying "intelligence." What can people mean when they refer to computers in this way?

Since these concepts involving the so-called mental aspects of machines are difficult to define by themselves or to account for in terms of more primitive concepts, there is a temptation to avoid the whole matter. One way of avoiding the issue is simply to declare that "intelligence" is a term that need not be limited to the discussion of humans alone. Another proposal, that intelligent may be appropriately used to describe the performance of any machine that, a century earlier, would have required human intellectual ability, would result in entire classes of simple machines (going back at least to the abacus) being regarded as intelligent.

Since we have so little understanding of what "thinking" is, either in terms of the processes involved or the physical mechanisms that support them, the question "Do computers think?" has been considered by some writers to be a vacuous one. Arguing that this would remain a vacuous question for an indefinite period of time, Alan M. Turing proposed an alternative procedure which he suggested could produce an answer, in principle at least. His proposal has since become known as the Turing Test. In one form of the test, we imagine having two teletype terminals; one is conected with an unseen human, and the other is connected to a computer. An interviewer, who does not know to which each teletype

is connected, is allowed to ask questions using the two teletypes
for a given length of time. He must then decide on the basis of the
observed responses which teletype is connected to the computer
and which is in communication with the human. If the interviewer
cannot successfully distinguish between them, then, Turing
argued, the computer could be said to be capable of thinking. Turing himself wrote:

> I believe that in about fifty year's time it will be possible to pro-
> gramme computers, with a storage capacity of about 10^9, to make
> them play the imitation game so well that an average interrogator
> will not have more than a 70% chance of making the correct identifi-
> cation after five minutes of questioning. The original question,
> "Can machines think?" I believe to be too meaningless to deserve
> discussion. [126]

This question and Turing's proposal for dealing with it raise difficult and subtle questions, which have been the subject of a great
deal of discussion since then.

In any case, "thinking" is a term that would seem to belong to
the vocabulary we use for the very highest-level descriptions of
people and perhaps some of the other higher animals. It is both
fuzzy and ambiguous, and includes many kinds of borderline situations. But would it under any conditions be appropriate to apply
it to plants, even though some do remarkable things, such as keeping their leaves turned toward the sun and capturing insects? Suppose we were asked to decide whether a particular object possessed
a "hunting skill," another fuzzy concept. We might declare that
this is a concept too meaningless to deserve discussion and instead
design a test for it. We could then proceed to compare the performance of a frog, a Venus's flytrap, and a piece of flypaper in
catching small insects. Suppose that over a period of five minutes
each of these caught 70 percent of the insects to which they were
exposed. Would we then conclude that these objects shared to the
same degree the high-level property "hunting skill"? I believe that
we know too much about these objects and their capabilities to be
comfortable with such a conclusion. But since not nearly as much
is known about "thinking," Turing's proposal, with its apparent
plausibility, has exerted a considerable appeal.

But let us return to the practical issues involved, and consider
the specific processes in which either computers or humans have

clear and distinct advantages. The more obvious advantages of computers stem directly from their hardware capabilities, and to a lesser degree from the programs that permit us to use these capabilities. Perhaps the most remarkable advantages of computers are the huge volumes of data they can store, and the speed and accuracy with which they can manipulate these data. These in turn derive from such technologies as materials science (semiconductors, ferromagnetism, plastics, cryogenics), circuit and system design (computer architecture), and fabrication techniques (integrated circuits). The rapid advances in these fields over the past two decades have made digital electronics, including computer engineering, one of the very few major technologies whose products have shown a precipitous and continuing decline in cost per unit of performance.

Since the introduction of the integrated circuit in about 1960. the cost per function of computers has decreased at a rate of nearly 50 percent each year, and this seems likely to continue over the near future. The result is that still greater data-storage capacity (per unit cost) will become available, and the economical storage of enormous data files in "knowledge" bases will become practicable. It should quite soon become possible, in principle, to store all the information in our hospital charts, in our medical libraries, and in the administrators' file cabinets in machine-readable form. However, the costs of converting all this information into such form would be staggering if we were limited to current manual data-entry methods. And how this information might then be usefully processed or otherwise utilized is another question for the future. Nevertheless, the promise of storing very large amounts of data, and of subsequently using it to advantage (both cheaply and rapidly), is perhaps the most attractive feature of computer technology. The present limitations to such efforts are perhaps associated less with the hardware limitations than with the lack of clear ideas as to what we would do with all these data, the costs of acquiring and entering data, uncertainties as to the best form in which the data should be represented and stored, and the limitations of current software for keeping track of them (data management systems).

The speed of computers when performing logic tasks is extremely rapid and, for the kinds of simple calculations we might otherwise do mentally or with a mechanical desk calculator, their performance is extraordinarily impressive. In processing physiological signals, or the outputs of most laboratory instruments, the computations can usually be performed in "real time" (the computations being completed at substantially the same rate at which the process is occurring) using small computers. In some nonarithmetical processing, the response may be equally rapid—say, in the retrieval and display of a patient's record—but with other programs, such as with image processing (e.g., computerized axial tomography, or CAT), natural-language processing systems, or with AI programs more generally, the response times may be inconveniently long. A more rapid response may always be obtained, of course, by using greater computing power, but only at an increased cost. The speed of processing depends on the hardware (both at the component level and in its architecture), the software, and on the means of encoding employed. Advances can be expected to be made on all fronts, though perhaps more impressively with hardware. Yet certain types of calculations are limited by issues of complexity. These inordinately complex calculations arise from a "combinatorial explosion," an unrestrained growth in the magnitude of certain kinds of computation, which will forever remain beyond the practical limits of computation. These limitations can be estimated from computability theory and the laws of physics, and they set limits *in principle* as to what can be calculated. Even though a problem may be formally shown to be computable, if the running time required for its solution on the most advanced computer conceivable is equal to the expected future life of the universe, it would hold little interest for us.[4]

Storage capacity and speed are the characteristics in which computers win hands down, *if* we can suitably formalize our applications and develop programs that can take advantage of them. Then there are other properties of computers, such as precision, which will be valuable in many applications but not necessarily so with all. When accuracy is purchased at the price of rigidity of performance, the cost may be too great for many high-level medical applications where quantitative precision is rarely needed. Finally, the reliability of computing systems, which may be achieved through the use of redundant components and subsystems, can be made arbitrarily great. Although parts of machines may wear out or fail, systems can be designed (as the mathematician John von Neumann has pointed out) that will not. Nor do they ever become tired or distracted.

The most important present limitation in the use of computers in medicine is the difficulty of finding suitable means for applying them directly to the solution of high-level problems. Computers necessarily operate in a formal way; the high-level processes in medicine (including much of judgment) are relatively informal ones. We noted at the end of the previous chapter that the development of higher-level programming languages might give the appearance of closing the gap between the rigidity and precision of the logic processes required at the machine level, and the informal and unstructured problems we find in the world. But as we saw, this does not appear to be the case.

When we consider such high-level clinical topics as disease, diagnosis, management of the patient, and inquiries into etiology, the formalization gap is extremely wide, though not uniformly so. Clinical topics do have their low-level features as well as high-level ones, and these can be dealt with individually and powerfully using low-level methods. But we cannot put the whole thing together and create unified descriptions without resorting to abstractions that permit us to reduce the formalization gap, and thus to be able to speak of such things as "pain" and "neurons" in the same breath.

What, then, are the peculiar capabilities of people which are not shared by computers, particularly as they are needed in processing information? We can enumerate some of them. Humans are always connected to the world about them by being *in* particular situations. These situations provide a continually changing environment (sets of contexts) within which human cognitive activities proceed. Humans know where they are, who they are and, to an appropriate degree, what is expected of them. Humans are also forever adapting, improving, and creating and, though driven by particular purposes, they may freely change their goals when novel circumstances arise. These capabilities have a great effect on the ways in which humans process information, and they circumscribe entire areas of information processing which, for years to come and perhaps indefinitely, will be reserved to people. Computers, so far, would seem to do none of these things to a significant degree. But humans are tool-using creatures, and even though many of our cognitive processes appear unlikely to be taken over by computers, it is almost surely the case that computer-based tools will be developed to assist in these purposes. We have perhaps not yet quite reached the stage at which our tools can amplify our cognitive processing to the dramatic extent that engines and machinery can extend our muscular powers. Yet we are fairly far along and have many aids to cognitive processing, including the tools already considered.

In addition, we have witnessed the development of such novel information technologies as computer graphics, which permit us to do entirely new kinds of things. The graphical display of complex macromolecular structures has reached a stage far beyond the representations possible with mechanical models [64]. The processing of radiographic data acquired through the CAT techniques now allow us to create images corresponding to arbitrary planes of section, and to manipulate these images in much the same way that molecular models or geometric forms can now be manipulated. There seems no reason why the same processes will not soon be applied to microscopic images, acquired at the levels of both optical and electron microscopy, and provide structural information about tissues and cells that is now denied us.

In the analysis of large quantities of data, where modern database management systems better meet the needs of the clinical investigator, we find another useful coming together of the characteristics of men and machines. Here the power of computer technology in manipulating huge volumes of data, and the human capability of introducing order into chaos by invoking relevance and by detecting "interesting" phenomena, form a combination in the most fruitful tradition of tool-use. This application is a fairly recent one in medicine. Few clinical data bases have so far been constructed that are both deep in detail and broad in coverage, or that are capable of enabling us to browse with convenience. Experience with such data bases that do exist has been relatively limited; any predictions one might make of their future impact upon medicine would almost surely fall short of the mark.

One of the application areas that has long been cited as having a particular need for such a tool is the study of chronic diseases. In the case of acute illnesses (most infectious diseases, trauma), the time lapse between cause and effect is short, and it is in these cases that the recognition of causation may be relatively easy. Chronic diseases, in contrast, may take such long periods of time to develop that the relations between cause and effect may be difficult to discern. The following example will illustrate this process. Suppose we have a small box with two externally visible features—a light bulb and a toggle switch. We might hand this to someone and ask him to find out and "explain" its behavior. After examining it briefly, he may casually flip the switch, whereupon the light would go on. When he restored the switch to its original position, the light would go out again. He may then rapidly move the switch back and forth and the lamp would follow by going on and off. The causal explanation of this behavior could be readily discovered by a child. But now let us introduce a complication: inside the box there is a time-delay mechanism, and in the previous experiment the time delay was set to zero. We now increase the time delay to one minute and repeat the above experiment with a different subject. Now when the switch is flipped on and off nothing seems to happen. Then a short time later, while the observer may be puzzling over what to do next, the lamp goes on for a moment, and then goes off. An adult subject might immediately recognize the connection between his previous manipulation of the switch and the subsequent behavior of the lamp, or this might not occur to him until later. The problem has now become more difficult. We could then go on and complicate matters further by increasing the time delay to an hour, a week, or to a decade. We can imagine the device having been studied by different observers, one after another for various periods of time, who may have recorded what they did to the device and described its responses. Finally, while in the possession of some later observer, who may have access to these records, the light begins to go on and off in some irregular manner. What are the chances of his being able to account for this behavior, given the evidence available to him? This last scenario is not unlike the case of a patient with a chronic disease for which the causes lie in the past. The earlier participants in the care of this patient, having had little in particular to look for, may have provided completely accurate descriptions of the patient, which will be of no use to their successors. And (equally likely) they may have treated the patient without recording exactly what they thought or did at the time.

There is no purely deductive solution to this problem, either with our thought-experiment or in actual clinical practice. We not only do not, but we cannot, systematically collect data to serve later purposes that cannot be anticipated. Nor can we simply attempt to record everything. The (probably) apocryphal story is told of an Englishman who, convinced that science progressed through observation, and being moved to contribute to this cause, devoted the remainder of his life to maintaining accurate and detailed records of everything he observed and did, and finally willed his accumulated collection to the Royal Society for their use! This simply doesn't work.

Our analogy of a light-box to the clinical situation fails, however, in one important respect. Vesalius and others have opened the box for us, and to the extent that they were able, described its contents. Their successors down to the present time have continued to extend these observations, and to devise increasingly effective descriptions and explanations. This knowledge has been incorporated into our current theories of medicine, which guide our observations. And unlike the mythical Englishman, we do not attempt to describe everything. If we cannot always know in advance exactly which features of our present patients will prove to be of the most importance, our intuition regarding what is relevant frequently puts us on the right track. But even this may leave us with enormous amounts of descriptive material to be recorded and later analyzed, and here technology can help us. We need all the help we can get in this difficult inductive process as we attempt to identify causes in chronic diseases, cancer, occupationally induced illnesses and, in general, in disorders with long periods of latency.

It seems likely that our most effective information systems for a long time to come will be combinations of men and machines. The machine will be increasingly employed as a sophisticated and powerful tool providing those characteristics of machines that can outperform humans, but operating under the direction of a human, who alone is likely to be able to identify problems worth solving, and who must decide when to use a machine and when to turn it off.

10.3 A Reintegration

Most of the account here has been occupied with the analysis, the taking apart, of informational and medical processes. Yet from the beginning we have stressed that medicine is concerned with wholes. The clinician's task, unlike that of the biochemist or the physiologist, ranges from the top to the bottom of the hierarchical scheme of nature. If, in order to account for some abnormal finding, the physician must explore matters at higher and lower levels, the task is not completed until all the data have been reassembled into a conceptual whole. Carrying this out effectively calls for a unique combination of skills and attitudes, and it is this combination of skills and attitudes that characterize the accomplished clinician.

In commenting upon the need for a broader perspective on illness, Eisenberg wrote:

> The image of the doctor as a technician contributes to the paradox of patients being dissatisfied at a time when the profession considers that its powers are at their greatest. We generate false expectations for cure that lead to malpractice suits when medical fallibility rather than personal incompetence is the issue. Virtuosity in performing too readily becomes an end in itself and blunts sensitivity to purpose. [34]

There is no point in resurrecting here the art versus science issue along the traditional lines, or repeating the endless cant about medical "holism." For one thing, we have never strayed far from this topic, although we have not addressed it systematically. We have emphasized a hierarchical perspective in which these questions can be seen in a somewhat different light, and which might provide the insight urged by Eisenberg. Our information model acknowledges that the pains and discomforts of a patient are high-level matters for which physicians increasingly seek lower-level explanations. We have seen, too, that the physician cannot emphasize any particular hierarchical level to the exclusion of all others. In an article on the patients' quality of life during the treatment of acute myeloid leukemia, P. S. Burge and coauthors comment:

> The present preoccupation with intensive therapy appears to blind physicians to the poor quality of life which their patients lead. The aim of treatment is too often to induce a haematological remission (an irrelevance to the patient) rather than to improve the quality of life. [20]

While a hematological remission is a low-level affair and the quality of life a high-level one, the oncologist might justly reply that without the former there will be little of the latter. And the oncologist may be just as aware of the importance of the quality of life as any physician. But no physician has quite the stake in the matter, nor the view of it, as the patient. It is when we think about patients only in terms of low-level attributes that we dehumanize the practice of medicine. The employment of technology has little to do with it, and dehumanization is done poorly by machines, though well by people.

To ensure humane medical care by keeping the patient's wholeness before our minds requires a degree of synthesis not called for in the sciences. Throughout the history of science, the attention of scientists and the content of their theories and laws have been concerned with nature taken at single, and usually low, levels. It is primarily during the last century that the conceptual contacts between hierarchical levels have become objects of interest in themselves, and only over the past few decades that such interlevel fields as chemical physics, quantum chemistry, and molecular biology have emerged. These newer subjects represent the organized probings in the hierarchy of nature in a vertical direction. Yet this undertaking has always been the lot of the clinician, whatever the state of knowledge has been.

Since the laws and theories of physical science have had this largely local relevance, and a concern focused primarily at single levels, their applicability to the synthetic problems of clinical medicine has been somewhat restricted. Scientific knowledge (especially physical science) has this laminated quality, and works best when applied horizontally. It follows that our application programs (our formal means of applying our knowledge) and our computations do likewise. Our ability to explain processes and to predict events by means of causal linkages proceeds most smoothly along particular levels. This is saying no more than that the laws of chemistry are more useful to us for predicting chemical outcomes than, say, for predicting the result of a presidential election.

By its nature, medicine finds itself in one sense at cross-purposes with science. Although the knowledge of medicine is enormously dependent upon the results of science, its purposes are different and, unless this is clearly seen, we invite endless confusion in attempting to distinguish one from the other. By being at "cross-purposes" I am in no way proposing that they are antithetical either in spirit or in their concern for truth, but only that they have different aims.

A useful insight into this point is provided by the contrast drawn by Daniel Schwartz and coworkers between the "explanatory" and the "pragmatic" attitudes in the design of clinical trials. An example of theirs makes the distinction clear [109, 110]. Suppose one wants to evaluate, by means of a clinical trial, the effectiveness of a new drug which is purported to act as a radiosensitizer in the radiation therapy of tumors. Suppose, too, that a treatment period of a month with the drug is required before the radiation therapy is begun. The design of a suitable clinical trial would include the need for a control group that would receive radiotherapy alone. The clinical experiment could then be conducted in two different ways. Patients could be randomly entered into either the treatment group and begin with the drug phase, or into the control group and undergo radiotherapy without first receiving the drug. This procedure would mean that, on average, the patients in the control group would be receiving radiation therapy one month earlier in the progression of their disease than patients in the experimental group, making the two groups different in this *additional* respect. In order to eliminate this difference and to make the two groups identical, except for the effect of the drug, an alternative procedure could be employed in which the radiation treatment of the control group would be withheld for a period of a month, thus restoring the theoretically desirable symmetry to the trial.

In analyzing these two protocols, the authors point out that, if we feel the purpose of the trial is to increase our knowledge of radiobiology, and if we wish to maximize our gain in explanatory power, the second procedure has the advantage. A physician taking the view that the second procedure was the "proper" protocol to use would be said to have what the authors call an "explanatory" attitude. An opposite view may be taken by the "pragmatists" who would argue that the justification for undertaking the trial is not so much to conduct an experiment in biology as to be able to devise an improved therapeutic procedure. This purpose can be accomplished just as well with the first protocol.

In practice, the choice between these protocols would probably depend on the risk entailed by withholding radiation therapy for a month in the control group, but information about this point would be difficult to obtain. An experiment to determine this directly would probably be unethical given that radiotherapy in this particular example is regarded as being helpful. The choice between these protocols would be made on the basis of an estimate of the risk involved in delaying treatment. A compromise might be reached by selecting the second protocol but shortening the drug pretreatment period from a month to, say, two weeks, thereby reducing the treatment delay of the controls. The authors go on to point out that such compromises will fail to satisfy anyone, and that they may be self-defeating as well. The trial may then fail to answer either the biological question or the pragmatic-clinical one, and it might better not be done at all.

The issue here may not be entirely an ethical one. Depending on the estimated risk in delaying treatment, and the promise of the experimental treatment, the importance of doing the biological experiment may prevail. But the difference between the explanatory and pragmatic attitudes is an important one, and it frequently helps in distinguishing between biological and clinical investigations. Neither procedure has a higher regard for the truth than the other, but one seeks explanation and the other improved treatment. These may be very different goals.

Much of the art versus science issue simply disappears when we analyze specific medical objects and processes, and allocate them to their appropriate hierarchical levels. We read, for example, that "...we must [in medicine] make a choice in communication between the freedom of the artist and the precision of the scientist" [42]. It would seem that we need not make such choices at all. In fact, it does not seem our choice to make. The difference lies not between choices, which we may readily exercise, but in the subject matter. We must "...look for precision in each class of things just so far as the nature of the subject admits." The continuing disclosure of the structure of the world has provided us with an improving perspective which was denied to Aristotle, and we must be willing to revise our ideas as to when precision is appropriate and when it is not. Nevertheless, the only means we have for talking about (even thinking about) man and disease is with the use of high-level, everyday terms and high-level descriptions, as well as low-level ones.

And that brings us back to our starting point, the matter of viewpoint. E. B. Wilson wrote in 1925:

> Life is an unbroken series of cell-divisions... it is a continuum, a never-ending stream of protoplasm.... The individual is but a passing eddy in the flow which vanishes and leaves no trace. [139]

A chemist might just as accurately observe that:

> Matter is an unbroken series of chemical changes . . . it is a continuum, a never-ending stream of oxidations, dissociations, combinations, and reductions. . . . Chemical identity is but a passing eddy in the history of a molecule which vanishes and leaves no trace.

And in this regress, the elementary particle physicist will have the last word. Yet who is to have the first? As physicians, we have a particular concern with human individuals, and we must grant that we cannot describe them effectively without talking about atoms and cells. But physicians know that they are expected to do more than that and, unlike chemists and biologists, they must examine the relations between all levels of existence. Medicine, in short, appears to be the enterprise offering us the greatest opportunity (and assigning us the heaviest of responsibilities) for describing the nature of man in all the interrelated levels of his complexity.

Notes

1: Theories of Information

1. Although equating information with "reduced uncertainty" has a plausible ring to it, if we go on and inquire what "uncertainty" is, we are usually told—you guessed it—that it is a lack of information. Such circular definitions are of little help to us. And what then is "disease"? "Well, that is an impaired state of health!"

2. Because the "information" sector of the economy is growing more rapidly than the GNP as a whole, this fraction was more recently estimated to be about 40%. For a recent review, see Daniel Bell, "The social framework of the information society," p. 163 in *The Computer Age: A Twenty Year Review,* eds. M. L. Dertouzos and J. Moses (Cambridge, Mass.: MIT Press, 1979).

3. Which came from Boltzmann's original entropy measure, and which, following Szilard's paper on Maxwell's demon ["Ueber die Entropieverminderung in einem thermodynamischen System bei Eingriffen intelligenter Wesen," *Zeit, fur Physik* (1929), 53:840-856] and Brillouin's referring to information as negative entropy (*Scientific Uncertainty and Information* [New York: Academic Press, 1964]) completed the link between "information" and thermodynamics.

The predictions of the 1950s and early 1960s that this new "information theory" would provide a deeper insight into human communications do not seem to have been fulfilled. We will consider one of these (Weaver's proposal) later in this chapter. For a more complete and fairly recent account of this matter, see Nauta, D., *The Meaning of Information* (The Hague-Paris: Mouton, 1972).

4. But see for example Simon [118] vs. Geschwind [46].

5. A somewhat similar concept was earlier proposed by K. R. Popper when he suggested that the information content of a proposition could be measured by the number of ways in which it might be falsified. A theory that claims more is more vulnerable to falsification and, therefore, contains more information. The logician Rudolf Carnap argued, in a similar way, that the information content of a proposition could be measured by the number of other propositions that it entailed.

2: Problems with "Information"

1. There are substantial differences between sentences and propositions (which is what Russell is writing about), and not all sentences or messages are concerned with facts. We will be mainly concerned here, however, with declarative sentences.

2. Ordinary utterances are always made in a situation, and will thus have a context. But written messages commonly occur in isolation; in writing the opening sentence of a novel or the first line of a poem the first and urgent task of the author is to begin to establish a context.

3. I am using the term *nominal* here simply as a less awkward equivalent for "nameable thing"; it is not intended to have any connotations beyond this.

4. We will be more concerned with information statements that correspond to *propositions* than to *sentences;* the difference between them being that the former will always have truth values (commonly they are either true or false), whereas the latter need not.

5. What we are here calling *complete* is analogous to a well-formed formula in the predicate calculus; the *information statement* is analogous to either a *closed sentence* or to a *proposition.*

6. These are the characteristic sounds heard by the physician with a stethoscope when there is consolidation in a patient's lungs.

7. This use of the term *open* is not to be confused with its use in the predicate calculus such as in "an open sentence," where it refers to what we have here considered to be a message fragment or predicate. An information statement is already complete; it will be considered open if further attributes can be added, and this will always be the case when describing natural objects or events.

8. It has been argued that the diameter, circumference, area, and perimeter are additional attributes. Since these are functionally dependent upon the radius, and therefore deducible from it, they add nothing to our description of C, and are tautological. However, depending upon one's point of view (see J. Lyons [74]) they, too, could be listed if desired, and the statement then closed.

9. A word will be considered to be *ambiguous* if it can be used to refer

to more than a single kind of thing. The word *pitcher* is used to refer to a type of container, and (in the United States) to a particular member of a baseball team. This distinction may be indicated orthographically by using *pitcher*$_1$ and *pitcher*$_2$. *Fuzziness* is a different notion. An attribute is fuzzy when membership in the indicated class occurs gradually rather than suddenly. The words *tall* and *short* are fuzzy, though perfectly clear. *Vagueness* is a different thing still. The word *table* is vague, although we ordinarily regard it as quite clear. We might think of our dining-room table as a standard or exemplar of what a table should be, in which case a proctoscopy table, or a crate used as a table on a camping trip, would be at some distance from the standard. When nominals or attributes are imprecise in this sense, we will employ the term "vague."

Words may be ambiguous, fuzzy, vague, all of these, or none of these. *Pitcher* is ambiguous and can mean *pitcher*$_1$ or *pitcher*$_2$, but *pitcher*$_1$ (a container) is vague, as well. There are some containers that are clearly "pitchers" (a cream pitcher), and others that are clearly not (a frying pan), but there are many spoutless containers that might be used as a cream pitcher and are close enough to cause trouble. The word *light* is also ambiguous; *light*$_1$ = not heavy, *light*$_2$ = not dark, and *light*$_3$ = an incandescent object or fixture. In its first two meanings it is fuzzy, and in its third, it is vague.

3: The Structure of Descriptions

1. I am here employing a "classical" view of atomic structure for simplicity. This will in no way prejudice our approach to the description of matter, as will be seen later. For the benefit of the reader who may be unfamiliar with these terms, it suffices to explain that they refer to physical attributes that are readily (if indirectly) measurable, and analogous to the attributes of ordinary, tangible objects. These are the *properties* of subatomic particles, just as size, color, and shape are properties of fruit.

2. In order to decide whether an attribute is *necessary* or not when establishing class membership, we require knowledge of only a particular kind of object. When we define a class, our definition establishes which attributes are *necessary*. *Sufficiency* is a far different matter, and requires knowledge about the rest of the world. If we are to claim that the finding of Koplik spots is sufficient for the diagnosis of measles, we must have certain knowledge that they occur in no other diseases. This means that we must have knowledge not just of measles but of *all* diseases. Beyond this, sufficient attributes may function singly in deciding class membership, whereas the conditions set for necessary attributes must be met as a whole.

3. What we are claiming is that a theory sufficient for the description

of a particular level (i.e., a complete theory for this level need not be capable of predicting properties that emerge at the next higher level. As such properties become known to us, we can then extend our theories of these levels to include them, and these modified theories serve as linking theories, which account for the properties extending across the interface between them.

4. What we are here recounting can be referred to a zero-order theory, and it is this one that will be considered throughout this book. For completeness however, the features of first- and second-order theories can be sketched. A first-order theory must deal explicitly with the problem of context, and the circumstance in which a nominal can take an attribute in one context and not in another, this being particularly so at higher hierarchical levels. Thus, grass is *not* green when it is dead, but only while flourishing, and we may state this:

$$(N \mid C_i \mid A) \text{ or (grass} \mid \text{actively growing} \mid \text{green)}$$

Similarly, to deal with ambiguity (again particularly so at higher levels), we must use a second-order theory, which is capable of handling multiple meanings. Either nominals or attributes may be ambiguous; is grass the stuff of which we make lawns, or marijuana? Is green a color or a judgment of unripeness? We can deal with this by keeping track of the various meanings which are involved:

$$(N_i \mid C_i \mid A_i)$$
(grass<lawn type> | actively growing | green<color>)

5. Because the structure of our descriptive statements may appear to reflect in some fundamental way the structure of the objects being described, there is a temptation to conjecture that our descriptions of such objects may be *isomorphic* with them. We need not go this far, in order to agree with A. J. Ayer that: "What we can establish is that [people's] experiences are similarly ordered. It is this similarity of structure that provides us with our common world: and it is only descriptions of this common world, that is, descriptions of structure, that we are able to communicate" [5].

6. This hierarchical feature of nature has been widely commented upon in recent years; for example by Herbert Simon, who employs the term *near-decomposability* [117], by Arthur Koestler in a commentary upon Simon's model [62], and by Jacob Bronowski [18].

7. See, for example, Alvin Feinstein's *Clinical Judgement,* pp. 381-384, for a thoroughgoing Comtean account of the relationships between medicine and the sciences.

8. Although Bronowski has argued in this connection that the cultural sources of language provide an artifactual component. (See Bronowski, J., "Human and Animal Languages," in *A Sense of the Future* (Cambridge, Mass.: MIT Press, 1977).

9. Named after Kurt Goedel, twentieth-century Austrian-American mathematician.

10. For example, the sentences "One and one are two," "One and two are three," can be extended indefinitely to produce a countably infinite set of different sentences. These sentences also happen to be true. But we can readily generate other infinite sets of sentences: "One and one are three," "One and one are four," and so on, which although untrue, are nevertheless propositions.

4: Information Processes

1. *Bergey's Manual of Determinative Bacteriology,* eds. R. E. Buchanan and N. E. Gibbons (Baltimore: The Williams and Wilkins Company, 1974).

2. The arbitrariness involved in the assignment of words to objects (in the attachment of meanings to words) seems first to have been emphasized by the Swiss linguist, Ferdinand de Saussure (1857-1913).

3. Michel Foucault attributes the motivation for his book *The Order of Things* (p. xv), New York: Random House, 1970 (*Les mots et les choses* [Paris: Editions Gallimard, 1966]) to his coming upon Borges's imaginative "quotation" from "a certain Chinese encyclopaedia" with its classification of animals: "(a) belonging to the Emperor, (b) embalmed, (c) tame, (d) sucking pigs, (e) sirens, (f) fabulous, (g) stray dogs, (h) included in the present classification, (i) frenzied, (j) innumerable, (k) drawn with a very fine camel hair brush, (l) *et cetera,* (m) having just broken the water pitcher, (n) that from a long way off look like flies."

4. One might speculate that chess may have forgotten origins as a practical "war game," or that Euclidean geometry developed from an earlier, perhaps Egyptian, empirical or "physical" geometry. Once games or mathematics have become rule-based or axiomatized, however, they are disconnected from the natural world, exist independently of it, and behave according to their rules and not the rules of the world. One cannot, therefore, hope to discover natural laws from the study of models of the world, unless the evidence for these laws has been carried over into the model during the process of abstraction. In constructing the models of physics, we have been particularly lucky, and this may have occurred because the required degree of abstraction is simply less. Until recent times, the creation and study of biological models has not been of comparable success. The most impressive of these have been those of molecu-

lar biology, subjects closer to physics than to biology. Even today it is necessary for biologists to work with the genuine articles.

5. Kelvin, of course, was speaking as a physicist, and in this context he was quite correct. The importance of measurability in physics had been recognized at least as far back as Pythagoras. In the life sciences, things are otherwise. Many laboratory tests in medicine can be carried out with reproducibility and precision, but they may not tell us much because of their low specificity (e.g., sedimentation rate, and the older liver-function tests, such as the thymol turbidity). Other tests, in contrast, which are entirely nonquantitative, may be highly specific, e.g., skin reactivity to injected antigens. The inverse of Kelvin's admonition, the implication that by measuring something we are on our way to understanding it, may be applied without insight and lead to all kinds of foolishness. Measurability seems most applicable and useful at lower descriptive levels before the fuzziness of attributes becomes too great. The measurement of high-level properties (e.g., in medicine or economics) can only be performed upon abstractions of these objects or processes, and may or may not be useful, depending upon how faithful or insightful the abstraction is.

6. I am indebted to Professor Otto Guttentag for drawing this example to my attention.

7. When we use "typical" in this context, we mean something quite different from "average." A microscope slide or an X-ray film chosen at random might be said to represent an "average" case but, for it to be typical or representative of some particular condition and to be the exemplar of a class, it must be selected with great care.

8. Whether the everyday world can be described in a language that does not use fuzzy terms seems to be one of the points of contention between the ordinary-language philosophers and the positivists.

9. From the point of view taken here, an atom is regarded as a simple object, although a layman might regard it as a complex one. A shoehorn, which might be taken to be a simple object is, in fact, a very complex one, as we have argued in section 3.3.

10. There is a limit to the precision that we can attain here, too, but this arises for a different reason—Heisenberg's Uncertainty Principle. The statistical view of nature expressed in quantum mechanics, though of particular relevance to the very small, applies to the large as well. The wave functions that describe how a silicon atom binds two oxygen atoms tell us something about the forces that hold mountains together, as well. But they cannot tell us all that we need to know about mountains, and we require the higher-level laws of geology and meteorology in order to do this. In these latter theories, the effect of the Uncertainty Principle becomes very diluted indeed.

11. The inapplicability of classical logic to what he has called "loose concepts," and to what we have regarded here as high-level nominals, has been discussed by Max Black [10].

12. In employing this term, it should not be inferred that we are embarking on a program of logical atomism. The term *primitive* is used here only in the sense of these being minimum statements, which just meet the completeness requirement as defined earlier.

13. We have not yet taken up the problem of introducing time into our information model. We could do so by explicitly including time as an attribute, and then write descriptive statements representing the state of affairs at t_1, t_2, t_3, ... etc., or by indicating that some attributes are time dependent. Or, we could proceed as is done in physics, by using continuous mathematics, and represent the time dependence of attributes by means of differential equations.

14. It is a matter of common experience that high-level descriptions often appear contradictory, even though they may be shown to be "true" individually. The problem here is not with "truth," but with "completeness." This is the origin of the "half-truth," a distinction well known to demagogues and advertisers, and a characteristic found in arguments that are limited to the length of a bumper sticker.

15. Consider the syllogism: (a) convicted thieves should serve prison terms, (b) John Doe is a convicted thief, therefore, (c) John Doe should be sentenced to prison. The reason we need law courts rather than algorithms as the basis for a criminal justice system is to be able to deal with such circumstances as John Doe being a thief because he stole a fire extinguisher from a store to extinguish the flames engulfing a loaded school bus.

5: Diseases

1. F. G. Crookshank, who provides the foregoing example (in an essay supplementary to C. K. Ogden and I. A. Richards, *The Meaning of Meaning,* 10th ed. (London: Routledge and Kegan Paul, 1949), has severely criticized the nominalist view, and has illustrated the confounding effect of reification upon the attempt to understand one particular disease, encephalitis.

2. Giovanni Battista Morgagni (1682-1771), founder of modern pathology.

3. *The International Classification of Diseases,* 9th rev., *Clinical Modification* (ICD-9-CM) (Ann Arbor, Mich.: Commission on Professional and Hospital Activities, 1978).

4. The difficulties raised by statistical definitions of disease have been

264 *Notes to Pages 104-126*

considered at some length by E. A. Murphy [88].

5. Sir Arthur Stanley Eddington (1882-1944), English astronomer and physicist.

6. For a contrary view of the ontology of mental illness, see G. L. Engel, *Science* (1977), 196: 129-136.

7. The question as to whether particular high-level attributes are "normal" or "abnormal" may become a normative one and subject to the influence of social and cultural processes. H. Fabrega has discussed these from an anthropological viewpoint [38].

8. For a recent discussion of Morgan's Canon and its application to the controversy of whether the foraging behavior of honeybees is to be attributed to a "dance-language" or to odor-sensing, see R. Rosin, (1980), "The Honey-Bee 'Dance Language' Hypothesis and the Foundations of Biology and Behavior," *Jour. Theor. Biol.* 87: 457-481. Although Morgan's Canon applies to phenomena that occur at high hierarchical (psychical) levels, its generalization to the entire set of hierarchical descriptions seems justified. It seems more parsimonious to seek explanations at lower levels than at higher ones, because hypotheses made at high levels contain large numbers of embedded attributes, are descriptively richer, and have a much greater information content. If we wish to be parsimonious, we want our hypotheses or assumptions to contain as little information as we can get by with.

9. Popper has discussed downward causation not only in the case of living organisms but with purely physical systems as well. His examples seem more convincing for the case of organisms than for nonliving systems, but the important question as to whether downward causation may be a distinctive property of living organisms remains an open one.

10. SNOP was developed by the American College of Pathology and the American College of Surgery, and was published in 1969.

11. SNOMED (Systematized Nomenclature of Medicine) was first published as a series of separate fascicles (Topography, September 1976; Morphology, September 1976; Etiology, September 1976; Function, September 1976; Disease, March 1977; Procedure, June 1977; and an Introduction, September 1977; Roger A. Cote, M.D., Editor-in-Chief) by the College of American Pathologists, Skokie, Illinois.

12. This linkage between ICD and SNOMED may be viewed as an enhancement of both, as in "[The] SNOMED disease field and [the] international classification of diseases: an imperative marriage of convenience," by C. Jeanty, and "The Advantages of augmenting the ICD code with SNOMED," by R. Thurmayr, papers given at the International Congress on Medical Informatics, Strasbourg, April 28-30, 1981 (4th Ann. Meeting, World Association of Medical Informatics). But this aug-

mentation is in coding capability alone, and neither system contains any medical knowledge (see below).

13. Our descriptions of CMIT refer to the 4th edition (1971), which succeeded earlier editions entitled *Current Medical Terminology*. A fifth edition appeared in early 1981.

6: The Processes of Diagnosis

1. This reasoning, as a means of distinguishing the two enterprises, has been criticized by Stephen Toulmin in *Evaluation and Explanation in the Biomedical Sciences,* eds. H. Tristram Engelhardt, Jr., and Stuart F. Spicker (Dordrecht: Reidel, 1975), pp. 51-66.

2. There are always conflicting factors that enter into this determination. Scheff has commented upon some of the consequences of the medical bias toward overdiagnosing disease rather that underdiagnosing it; that is, the preference of physicians in accepting Neyman's type (2) error (treating a patient who is actually well) rather than committing a type (1) error (ignoring a patient who is actually sick). See T. J. Scheff, "Decision rules, types of errors, and their consequences in medical diagnosis," *Behavior. Sci.* (1963), 8: 97-107. It should be noted that this was written before the medical malpractice "crisis" of the mid-1970s. The effect of this latter factor as an additional source of bias in the diagnostic process in favor of type (2) errors had not been taken into account by Scheff.

3. Polanyi has pointed out that the dynamical problem of maintaining balance on a bicycle involves following slightly curved paths in which, for a given angle of unbalance, the curvature of the path necessary to restore balance is inversely proportional to the square of the speed. But surely no one, he goes on, would claim on these grounds that a rider manages to remain upright by continuously solving this equation [97].

4. The distinction between "monothetic" and "polythetic" is attributed by Sokal to M. Beckner, in *The Biological Way of Thought* (New York: Columbia University Press, 1959), who originally used the terms *monotypic* and *polytypic*.

5. In deciding whether patients do, in fact, have the same disease (in order that their disease descriptions can be aggregated in this manner), the greatest authority has historically been accorded to the anatomical pathologist. Increasingly this may be decided upon the evidence of specialized laboratory testing involving many other disciplines, and concerning still lower-level attributes.

The reader will note the essential circularity of this process: patients are grouped on the basis of their resemblance; their common illness is named; and then this illness is characterized in terms of the same attributes that were employed in forming the patient aggregate. As a result, classification itself cannot have explanatory power.

6. Qualitative statements like these, with their use of "frequently," "may have," or "possibly," emphasize the softness of much of our medical knowledge. In the effort to make this knowledge more quantitative, such terms can, in principle, be replaced with empirically determined likelihoods. The probability that a patient having disease D will display attribute A_1, is spoken of as a conditional probability, and is written as $P(A_i \mid D)$. These conditional probabilities can be determined from clinical records, and they have been employed in various diagnostic programs.

7. Feinstein has distinguished between *pathogenetic* inference, in which one reasons from cause to effect, and *diagnostic* reasoning, which proceeds oppositely (Alvin R. Feinstein, "An analysis of diagnostic reasoning," *Yale Jour. Biol. and Med.* (1973), 46: 212-232). We have already called these the directions of *causality* and *explanation*, respectively.

8. The answer to Pauker's question is easily seen by a simple enumeration. With an incidence of 1 in 1,000, of a million women, 1,000 would have cancer and 999,000 would not. Of the 1,000 with cancer, 950 would give a true positive test result (sensitivity = 95%). Of the 999,000 women without cancer, 99,900 would give false positive test results (specificity = 90%) so that the total number of positive tests (both true and false positive) would be (950 + 99,900) or 100,850. But of the latter, only 950, or 0.9%, would actually have cancer (950/100,850), so that the probability of our single patient having breast cancer, given the positive test result, is less than 1%.

9. Predictive value of a positive test = [true positives/(true positives + false positives)] × 100.

7: The Clinical Process

1. I will employ the term *judgment* to include the collection of informal and intuitive decision processes which we use in the absence of explicit formulas or rules.

2. This metaphor is not unrelated to the one given in section 3.2 with respect to hierarchical levels. Here, however, we are concerned with a process; with a structure that is changing over time.

3. We will consider a problem to be well structured when it is *complete* (no *essential* information is missing) and *closed* (the solution is a member of the given solution set; the ideal differential diagnosis would be in the present context). Under this definition, few of the everyday problems of medicine would be regarded as well structured. The medical imperative,

however, commonly requires that a decision be made or an action initiated, on the basis of *partial* or *incomplete* information.

4. The most ambitious of these programs, INTERNIST, which selects from a set of several hundred medical disorders, would stand slightly to the left of the others, if they were represented in figure 7.1, but would still stand well to the right of point (A).

5. Pauker et al., estimated that the core knowledge of internal medicine might involve a million "facts," and that if the medical subspecialties were included, this might rise to two million [93].

6. The differences between point (A) and (B) applications serve as a demarcation between two types of artificial intelligence research. The second, and empirically the more successful kind, are increasingly being described by Edward Feigenbaum's term, *knowledge engineering*.

7. Before this attempt at putting microworlds together to form a world (like assembling jigsaw-puzzle pieces) becomes plausible, it will be necessary to demonstrate a procedure for taking apart descriptions of the world in such a way that pieces of this kind would result. This remains to be accomplished, and would appear a doubtful undertaking.

8. Among the various attributes of intelligence, the ability to deal with the novel would seem to rank high. Every day we (including young children) understand sentences that we have never heard before. We also understand new words whose meanings are never explicitly defined for us, but which we readily infer from the context. Unless we were capable of doing this, ordinary language acquisition would be impossible.

9. For a highly readable and informal account of the development of AI, the reader is referred to Pamela McCorduck's sympathetic review [77].

10. Physicians' preference for computer applications have, according to one recent survey, been ranked as follows (in decreasing order of interest): billing, accounting, medical records, word processing, literature file, insurance billing, computer-assisted instruction, data base applications, research laboratory applications, appointment scheduling, statistics, computer-aided diagnostics, patient history, control system, medical testing, inventory, drug interaction, practice survey, medical simulations, intensive-care monitoring, payroll, epidemiology, emergency room, and health-hazard appraisals (reported in *Computers and Medicine*, IX, 2 (Amer. Med. Assoc., 1980).

11. MEDLINE is the name given to a collection of data bases and retrieval programs that can be accessed remotely. It is maintained by the National Library of Medicine.

12. It is interesting to realize that we are on the threshold of a remarkable procedural change in the use of recorded knowledge. From medieval manuscripts to our present printed books, it has been the producers' and

users' implicit understanding that substantially the entire document would be read (used). When the time comes that we are able to store (and index) an entire medical library, including journals, on a few video disks, and have these at our fingertips in our offices and homes, it will be with the understanding that most of this material will never be read by us. Rather, it will be used as the source of *particular* information or data, which appropriate search methods would locate for us.

13. Homer R. Warner [131] has suggested the usefulness of making this connection, and Martin N. Epstein and Eric B. Kaplan [37] have conceptualized a framework in which this might be carried out. More recently, Robert Blum has described a program, RX, which uses this approach [15].

8: The Creation of Medical Information

1. The features of this activity that I have referred to as "monitoring" have been discussed by Churchman in relation to a number of classical models of cognition, and for this mental function he has used the term *the executive*. This knowing about our knowledge could just as well be called metaknowledge.

2. Zadeh has called such questions as these "surrogate questions." In creating surrogate questions, we follow the advice given by George Polya for problem solving: "If you cannot solve the proposed problem try to solve first some related problems. Could you imagine a more accessible related problem? A more general problem? A more special problem? An analogous problem? Could you solve a part of the problem?" [98].

3. In working with Jack Meyers on the INTERNIST project, Harry Pople reported a similar experience. Dr. Meyers appeared to be uncomfortable in attempting to recall and articulate his diagnostic reasoning process when discussing hypothetical cases in the abstract. Yet, in a clinical setting and when faced with an actual case, Dr. Meyers's attempts at introspection were more successful, even when the same processes were involved.

These experiences call to mind a phenomenon reported by de Groot in his studies with chess players. Experiments were conducted by arranging chess pieces in apparent mid-game positions. Some of these board positions were taken from unpublished, but actually played, games; the others were set up haphazardly, though in legal positions. Chess masters and novices were then shown these board positions briefly, and a short time later they were asked to reconstruct them from memory. The results showed that the masters' accuracy of recall was markedly superior to that of the novices in the case of the real-game positions, but that the two groups performed about equally in the case of the fictitious positions.

(A. D. de Groot, *Thought and Choice in Chess* (The Hague: Mouton, 1965). Our comprehension of situations seems to include an ability to distinguish between the natural and the artificial, and the questions we ask in actual situations have a different character from those we attempt to create in the abstract.

4. We formally defined "words" as alphanumeric strings preceded by a space and terminated by a comma, semicolon, or period. As a result of this definition, the sequence *21 to 50* would be treated as three 2-letter words. This definition, although yielding a few odd words such as *p* (from *p wave*), has in our experience been a satisfactory one.

5. As a passing comment upon the "soft" nature of high-level medical knowledge, it is interesting to note that, in CMIT, the word *possibly* occurs 2,405 times, *never* occurs 12 times, and *always,* 21 times.

6. This, of course, is a pure Hartley-Shannon theory concept, which is justified in this case by the "closed" character of CMIT. That is, there are a fixed number of named diseases described in the book. (However, this set of diseases is probably larger than the average physician can readily recall.)

7. The actual formula used for this is $S = 1 - (n/3262)$, where S is the specificity, and n is the number of diseases in which the attribute is mentioned.

8. The entropy formula we used was:

$$S_p(w) = -\sum_{i=0}^{10} p_i(w) \ln p_i(w)$$

$$p_i(w) = \frac{\dfrac{d_i(w) + 1}{d_i}}{\displaystyle\sum_{i=0}^{10} \dfrac{d_i(w) + 1}{d_i}}$$

$d_i(w)$ is the number of disease descriptions in which word *W* occurs at least once and which are assigned to category *i*.

9. All of the programs used in the studies of CMIT including RECONSIDER were written by my colleague David Sherertz whose contributions to this work were indispensable.

10. By this time, the program had been provided with a modest synonymy capability. My colleagues Rodney Ludwig, M.D., and Hyo Kim, M.D., constructed a synonym dictionary of some 3,000 medical terms so that if a particular term had been employed in a disease description and a synonym of that term were entered, a proper match would ensue.

11. Gerald Salton recently reviewed the problem of information re-

trieval, and summarized various methods that have been employed (*Computer,* Sept. 1980, 41-56). Among these methods is the use of pre-assigned weights used in much the same manner as we have used selection powers. T. E. Doskoscz has described a document-retrieval program for use with the MEDLINE data bases which uses a measure of "selection power" similar to the one described here [29].

12. In doing so we risk disregarding something important. As the average age of the population continues to increase, we will be finding increasing numbers of both multisystem diseases and instances of multiple diseases, and an obvious means of detecting the latter is through the recognition of attributes that do not readily cluster with the others.

13. With only a thousand different attributes, we can form 1,000 × 999 attribute pairs, but since the order is unimportant ("nausea" and "vomiting" being no different from "vomiting" and "nausea") this number is reduced by half, leaving about half a million. Important attribute clusters are of course not limited to pairs (e.g., "polydipsia," "polyphagia," and "polyuria"), and the combinations quickly number many millions.

14. A number of examples of word pairs of this type, which we called "Hong Kong" words, and object-modifier pairs (e.g., "erythroid-marrow") were mentioned in a paper delivered at the annual meeting of the Association for Computational Linguistics in 1980 [13].

15. Bayes' formula deals with the problem of inverting a probability, of computing the probability of $P(A|B)$ when $P(B|A)$ is known. Being able to perform this inversion allows one to use a knowledge of the observed past frequencies of events, to estimate their future likelihoods, and has been proposed as a basis of inductive inference.

9: The Representation of Medical Information

1. MACSYMA is a program for solving word problems. It has a limited natural-language capability, and is intended to solve arithmetic problems that are expressed in natural language rather than in the form of equations.

2. This need was recognized some years ago by the National Library of Medicine, which instituted a program of grants to support graduate and postgraduate training in the application of computers to medicine. These grants have resulted in the establishment of several such academic programs in the United States.

10: On the Proper Use of Men and Machines

1. We reluctantly continue the conventional practice of contrasting a computerized process with a "manual" one, although *hands* clearly have little to do with the things for which we ordinarily use computers.

2. The experiences with a very early medical order-entry system implemented on a ward at the Massachusetts General Hospital, and intended for use by the house staff, seems to have been the basis for this assumption. Considering that the terminals used were noisy mechanical ones (like teletype machines), that the motivation behind the project lay with the computer engineers and system developers, that the system itself offered few rewards for the medical staff or patients, and that operating the system involved extra duty for the always busy house staff (since it took more time than the conventional manual system), it is small wonder that users' reactions were generally negative. Yet the generalizations made about this experience, though negative, involve entirely different aspects of the experiment: It was said that physicians will not type because (a) by and large they are not skilled at this activity (which is probably true), and (b) that they would regard this as being "secretarial" in nature and hence beneath their dignity! (Which is speculation.) This point of view quickly became dogma among medical information system designers, and to this day no commercial MIS has been designed in the expectation that a physician would utilize a keyboard in using the system. I would wager that, if a medical computing system were to become available that offered a *significant* professional benefit to physicians (and which, for whatever reasons, required him to operate its keyboard personally or forego its benefits), typing courses would quickly become the most popular continuing medical education activity! This particular problem may be self-limiting, of course, as increasing numbers of medical students become familiar with typewriters, and computers as well.

3. El Camino Hospital, Mountain View, California.

4. The ultimate hardware limitations can be stated in purely physical terms. One cannot propagate signals faster than the velocity of light, build components smaller or more closely spaced than the sizes of elementary particles, nor employ more of them than there are elementary particles in the universe. Although present technology is nowhere near the latter two of these limits, there are well-defined classes of problems that are noncomputable because of them. We are not, however, similarly able to set limits upon what can be accomplished through different methods of data representation or data processing because of the lack of the necessary general theories.

References

1. American Medical Association. 1952. *Systematized Nomenclature of Disease and Operations*. Chicago.
2. ———. 1971. *Current Medical Information and Terminology*. Edited by B. Gordon. Chicago.
3. Auerbach, I. 1974. Future developments in data processing. *Information Science: Search for Identity*. Edited by A. Debons. New York: Marcel Dekker (pp. 215-220).
4. Augustine. *The Confessions of St. Augustine Book I, Ch. 8*. Translated by R. Warner. New York: Mentor, 1963.
5. Ayer, A. J. 1956. *The Problem of Knowledge*. Middlesex, England: Hammondsworth.
6. Bar-Hillel, Y. 1964. *Language and Information*. Boston: Addison-Wesley.
7. Barnett, G. O. The modular Hospital Information System. *Computers and Biomedical Research*. Vol. 4. Edited by R. W. Stacy and B. D. Waxman. New York: Academic Press.
8. Belkin, N. J. 1978. Information concepts for information science. *Jour. of Documentation* 34: 55-85.
9. Berlinski, D. 1976. *On Systems Analysis: An Essay Concerning the Limitations of Some Mathematical Methods in the Social, Political, and Biological Sciences*. Cambridge, Mass.: MIT Press.
10. Black, M. 1970. *Margins of Precision: Essays in Logic and Language*. Ithaca, N.Y.: Cornell University Press.
11. Bleich, H. L. 1969. Computer evaluation of acid-base disorders. *Jour. Clin. Invest.* 48: 1689-1696.
12. ———. 1972. Computer-based consultation: electrolyte and acid-base disorders. *Amer. Jour. Med.* 53: 285-291.

13. Blois, M. S., D. D. Sherertz, and M. S. Tuttle. 1980. Word and object in disease descriptions. *Proc. of the 18th Ann. Meeting Assoc. for Computational Linguistics.* A.C.L.

14. Blois, M. S., and R. R. Henley. 1971. Strategies in the planning of medical information systems. *Journées d'Informatique Médicale,* Paris: IRIA, 1971.

15. Blum, R. 1982. *Discovery and Representation of Causal Relationships from a Large Time-Oriented Clinical Database: The RX Project.* New York: Springer Verlag.

16. Boden, M. A. 1977. *Artificial Intelligence and Natural Man.* New York: Basic Books.

17. Bolinger, R. E., and P. Ahlers. 1975. The science of 'pattern recognition.' *Jour. Am. Med. Assoc.* 233: 1289-1290.

18. Bronowski, J. 1970. New concepts in the evolution of complexity. *A Sense of the Future.* Cambridge, Mass.: MIT Press.

19. Buchanan, B. G., and E. A. Feigenbaum. 1978. Dendral and Metadendral: their applications dimension. *Artificial Intelligence.* 11: 5-24.

20. Burge, P. S., et al. 1975. Quality and quantity of survival in acute myeloid leukaemia. *Lancet.* 2: 621-624.

21. Cherry, C. 1957. *On Human Communication.* Cambridge, Mass.: MIT Press.

22. Chomsky, N. 1959. A review of B. F. Skinner's 'Verbal Behavior.' *Language.* 35: 26-58.

23. Churchman, C. W. 1971. *The Design of Inquiring Systems: Basic Concepts of Systems and Organization.* New York: Basic Books.

24. Cohen, H. 1960. The evolution of the concept of disease. *Concepts of Medicine.* Edited by B. Luch. Oxford University Press.

25. Collen, M. F., ed. 1974. *Hospital Computer Systems.* New York: John Wiley & Sons.

26. Commission on Professional and Hospital Activities. 1978. *The International Classification of Diseases* (*9th rev.*), *Clinical Modifications.* Ann Arbor.

27. Crooks, J., I. P. C. Murray, and E. J. Wayne. 1959. Statistical methods applied to the clinical diagnosis of thyrotoxicosis. *Quart. Jour. Med.* 28: 211-234.

28. DeDombal, F. T., D. J. Leaper, J. R. Staniland, A. P. McCann, and J. C. Horrocks. 1972. Computer-aided diagnosis of acute abdominal pain. *Brit. Med. Jour.* 2: 9-13.

29. Dosckosz, T. E. 1980. An associative interactive dictionary (AID) for online bibliographic searching. *Proc. ASIS.* 115: 105-109.

30. Dreyfus, H. L. 1979. *What Computers Can't Do, The Limits of Artificial Intelligence* (rev. ed.). New York: Harper Colophon Books.

31. Dudley, H. A. F. 1968. Pay-off, heuristics, and pattern recognition in the diagnostic process. *Lancet*. 723-726.

32. Durham, R. H. 1960. *Encyclopedia of Medical Syndromes*. New York: Hoeber.

33. Eddington, A. 1927. *The Nature of the Physical World*. London: Everyman's.

34. Eisenberg, L. 1977. Disease and illness. *Culture, Medicine and Society*. 1: 9-23.

35. Elstein, A. S., L. S. Shulman, and S. A. Sprafka. 1978. *Medical Problem Solving: An Analysis of Clinical Reasoning*. Cambridge, Mass.: Harvard University Press.

36. Engle, R. L., and B. J. Davis. 1963. Medical diagnosis: present, past and future. *Arch. Int. Med*. 112: 512-519.

37. Epstein, M. N., and E. B. Kaplan. 1977. Criteria for clinical decision making. *Computational Linguistics in Medicine*. Edited by W. Schneider and A.-L. Sagvall Hein. Amsterdam: North-Holland.

38. Fabrega, H. 1976. Toward a theory of human disease. *Jour. Nerv. and Mental Dis*. 162: 299-312.

39. Findlay, J. 1952. Goedelian sentences, a non-numerical approach. *Mind*. 51: 259-265.

40. Fitzgerald, L. T., J. E. Overall, and C. M. Williams. 1966. A computer program for diagnosis of thyroid disease. *Amer. Jour. Roent. Radium Ther. Nucl. Med*. 97: 901-905.

41. Fries, J. F., D. J. McShane, A. Harlow, and R. Kraines. TOD: a software system for the ARAMIS data bank. *Computer*. 12 (No. 11): 34-40.

42. Gabrielli, E. R., ed. 1972. *Clinically Oriented Documentation of Laboratory Data*. New York: Academic Press.

43. Galen, R. S., and S. R. Gambino. 1975. *Beyond Normality: The Predictive Value and Efficiency of Medical Diagnoses*. New York: John Wiley & Sons.

44. Garfield, S. 1974. *The Computer and New Health Care Systems*. In *Hospital Computer Systems*. Edited by M. F. Collen. New York: John Wiley & Sons.

45. Garner, W. R. 1962. *Uncertainty and Structure as Psychological Concepts*. New York: John Wiley & Sons.

46. Geschwind, N. 1981. Neurological knowledge and complex behaviors. *Perspectives on Cognitive Science*. Edited by D. A. Norman. Hillsdale, N.J.: Lawrence Erlbaum Associates.

47. Giebink, G. A., and L. L. Hurst. 1975. In *Computer Projects in Health Care*. Ann Arbor, Mich.: Health Administration Press.

48. Gorry, G. A. 1973. Computer-assisted clinical decision making. *Meth. Infor. Med*. 12: 45-51.

49. Gorry, G. A., H. Silverman, and S. G. Pauker. 1978. Capturing

clinical expertise: a computer program that considers clinical responses to digitalis. *Amer. J. Med.* 64: 452-460.

50. Graitson, M. 1981. Comments on the semantic classification of SNOMED. *Proc. of World Assoc. on Medical Informatics.* Strasbourg.

51. Grossman, J. H., G. O. Barnett, and M. T. McGuire. 1971. Evaluation of computer acquired patient histories. *Jour. Amer. Med. Assoc.* 215: 1286-1291.

52. Hamill, K. A., and A. Zamora. 1980. Use of titles for automatic document classification. *Jour. Amer. Soc. Inf. Sci.* 31: 396-402.

53. Hamilton, E. 1930. *The Greek Way.* New York: W. W. Norton.

54. Hampton, J. R., M. J. G. Harrison, J. R. A. Mitchell, et al. 1975. Relative contributions of history-taking, physical examination, and laboratory investigation to diagnosis and management of medical outpatients. *Brit. Med. Jour.* 2: 486-489.

55. Hargraves, M. M., H. Richmond, and R. Morton. 1948. *Proc. Staff Meeting, Mayo Clinic.* 23: 25-28.

56. Harris, Z. 1976. A theory of language structure. *Amer. Phil. Quart.* 13: 237-255.

57. Hartley, R. V. L. 1928. Transmission of information. *Bell Sys. Tech. Jour.* 7: 535.

58. Hebb, D. O. 1961. *Sensory Deprivation.* Cambridge, Mass.: Harvard University Press.

59. Henley, R. R., G. Wiederhold, et al. 1975. *An Analysis of Automated Record Systems: Vol. I,* and *Background Material: Vol. II.* University of California, San Francisco: Laboratory of Medical Information Science.

60. Jaki, S. L. 1969. *Brain, Mind, and Computers.* South Bend, Ind.: Gateway Editions Ltd.

61. Jelliffe, R. W., J. Buell, and R. Kalaba. 1972. Reduction of digitalis toxicity by computer assisted glycoside dosage regimens. *Ann. Int. Med.* 77: 891-906.

62. Koestler, A. 1967. *The Ghost in the Machine.* London: Hutchinson.

63. Kuepfmueller, K. 1924. Ueber Einschwingvorgaenge in Wellenfiltern. *Elek. Nach. Tech.* 1: 141.

64. Langridge, R., T. E. Ferrin, I. D. Kuntz, and M. L. Connolly. 1981. Real-time color graphics in studies of molecular interactions. *Science.* 211: 661-666.

65. Lapage, S. P., S. Bascomb, W. R. Willcox, and M. A. Curtis. 1973. Identification of bacteria by computer: general aspects and perspectives. *Jour. Gen. Microbiology.* 77: 273-290.

66. Ledley, R. S., and L. B. Lusted. 1959. Reasoning foundations of medical diagnosis. *Science.* 130: 9-21.

67. Lewis, T. 1980. Notes of a biology watcher, on artificial intelligence.

New Eng. Jour. Med. 302: 506-508.

68. Lewontin, R. C. 1978. Adaptation. *Sci. Amer.* 239: 215.
69. Library Association, The. 1969. *Classification and Information Control.* London.
70. Lindberg, D. A. B. 1979. *The Growth of Medical Information Systems in the United States.* Lexington, Mass.: Lexington Books/ D. C. Heath Company.
71. Linfors, E. W., and F. A. Nelson. 1980. The case for bedside rounds. *New Eng. Jour. Med.* 303: 1230-1233.
72. Lloyd, G. E. R. 1970. *Early Greek Science; Thales to Aristotle.* London: Chatto and Windus.
73. Lucas, R. W., W. I. Card, R. P. Knill-Jones, et al. 1976. Computer interrogation of patients. *Brit. Med. Jour.* 2: 623-625.
74. Lyons, J. 1977. *Semantics, Volume I.* Cambridge, England: Cambridge University Press.
75. Machlup, F. 1962. *The Production and Distribution of Knowledge in the United States.* Princeton, N. J.: Princeton University Press.
76. Mayne, J. G., M. J. Martin, W. F. Taylor, et al. 1972. A health questionnaire based on paper-and-pencil medium, individualized and produced by computer. *Ann. Int. Med.* 76: 923-930.
77. McCorduck, P. 1979. *Machines Who Think.* San Francisco: Freeman.
78. McKay, D. M. 1969. *Information, Mechanism and Meaning.* Cambridge, Mass.: MIT Press.
79. Medawar, P. 1977. "Emergence." In *The Fontana Dictionary of Modern Thought.* London: Fontana/Collins.
80. Meehl, P. E. 1954. *Clinical versus Statistical Prediction: A Theoretical Analysis and a Review of the Evidence.* Minneapolis: University of Minnesota Press.
81. ———. 1973. *Psychodiagnosis: Selected Papers.* Minneapolis: University of Minnesota Press.
82. Meyer-Steinig, T., and K. Sudhoff. 1928. *Geschichte der Medezin in Ueberblink mit Abbildungen.* Jena: Fischer.
83. Miller, G. A., and P. N. Johnson-Laird. 1976. *Language and Perception.* Cambridge, Mass.: Harvard University Press (p. 601).
84. Miller, R. A., H. E. Pople, Jr., and J. D. Myers. 1982. INTERNIST-I, an experimental computer-based diagnostic consultant for general internal medicine. *New Eng. Jour. Med.* 307: 468-476.
85. Minsky, M. 1969. Semantic Information Processing. Cambridge, Mass.: MIT Press.
86. Mitchell, T. M. 1977. Version spaces: a candidate elimination approach to rule learning. *Proc. International Joint Conf. on Artificial Intelligence.*
87. Morgan, C. O. 1900. *Animal Behavior.* London: Edward Arnold.

88. Murphy, E. A. 1976. *The Logic of Medicine*. Baltimore: The Johns Hopkins University Press.
89. Myers, J. D. 1980. Lecture at Symposium on Computer Applications in Medical Care. Washington, D.C.
90. Nagel, E. 1961. The Structure of Science. *Problems in the Logic of Scientific Explanation*. London: Routledge and Kegan Paul.
91. Nyquist, H. 1924. Certain factors affecting telegraph speed. *Bell Sys. Tech. Jour.* 3: 324.
92. Pauker, S. G. 1980. From a presentation at Symposium on Computers in Medicine: Applications of Artificial Intelligence Techniques. Stanford, Ca.
93. Pauker, S. G., G. A. Gorry, J. P. Kassirer, and W. B. Schwartz. 1976. Towards the simulation of clinical cognition: taking a present illness by computer. *Amer. Jour. Med.* 60: 981-996.
94. Peirce, C. S. 1931. *Collected Papers of Charles Sanders Peirce.* 8 vols., vol. ii. Edited by C. Hartshorne, P. Weiss, and A. Burks. Cambridge, Mass.: Harvard University Press.
95. Plato. *Timaeus and Critias.* Translated by Desmond Lee. Middlesex, England: Penguin, 1971.
96. Platt, J. R. 1964. Strong inference. *Science.* 146: 347-353.
97. Polanyi, M. 1958. *Personal Knowledge.* London: Routledge and Kegan Paul.
98. Polya, G. 1945. *How to Solve It.* Princeton, N.J.: Princeton University Press.
99. Popper, K. R. 1959. *The Logic of Scientific Discovery.* London: Hutchinson.
100. ———. 1972. *Objective Knowledge.* Oxford: Clarendon Press.
101. Quine, W. V. O. 1960. *Word and Object.* Cambridge, Mass.: MIT Press.
102. Rumelhart. D. E. 1981. *Understanding Understanding.* San Diego: Center for Human Information Processing, University of California.
103. Russell, B. 1940. *An Inquiry into Meaning and Truth.* London: Allen and Unwin.
104. ———. 1946. *History of Western Philosophy.* London: Allen and Unwin.
105. Ryle, G. 1954. *Dilemmas.* Cambridge, England: Cambridge University Press.
106. Rypka, E. W. 1980. Personal communication, and Johnson, L., Earton, L., and Rypka, E. W., 1979. The clustering of hemophilus species for purpose of identification. *Jour. Infect. Diseases.*
107. Saito, Masao. 1980. What have we gained through experience? *Medical Informatics.* 5: 107-109.

108. Schank, R. C. 1975. *Conceptual Information Processing*. Amsterdam: North Holland.
109. Schwartz, D., and J. Lellouch. 1967. Explanatory and pragmatic attitudes in clinical trials. *Jour. Chrn. Dis.* 20: 637-648.
110. Schwartz, D., R. Flamant, and J. Lellouch. 1970. L'essai therapeutique chez l'homme. *Clinical Trials*. Paris: Flammarion.
111. Scriven, M. 1979. "Clinical judgment." In *Clinical Judgment: A Critical Appraisal*. Edited by Englehardt, Jr., H. T., S. F. Spicker, and B. Towers. Holland: Dordrecht.
112. Shannon, C. E. 1948. The mathematical theory of communications. *Bell Sys. Tech. Jour.* 27: 379-423.
113. ———. 1965. Information Theory. *Encyclopedia Britannica*. 12: 245-246.
114. Shannon, C. E., and W. Weaver. 1949. *The Mathematical Theory of Communication*. Urbana, Ill.: University of Illinois Press.
115. Shortliffe, E. H. 1976. *Computer-Based Medical Consultations: MYCIN*. New York: Elsevier.
116. Shortliffe, E. H., B. G. Buchanan, and E. A. Feigenbaum. 1979. Knowledge engineering for medical decision making: a review of computer-based clinical decision aids. *Proc. IEEE.* 67: 1207-1224.
117. Simon, H. E. 1962. The architecture of complexity. *Proc. Amer. Phil. Soc.* 106: 467-482. (Reprinted in Simon, the Sciences of the Artificial, Cambridge, Mass.: MIT Press, 1969.)
118. ———. 1981. Cognitive science: the newest science of the artificial. *Perspectives on Cognitive Science*. Edited by D. A. Norman. Hillsdale, N.Y.: Lawrence Erlbaum Associates.
119. Slack, W. V., G. P. Hicks, and C. E. Reed. 1966. A computer-based medical history system. *New Eng. Jour. Med.* 247: 194-198.
120. Sneath, P. H. A. 1964. New approaches to bacterial taxonomy: use of computers. *Ann. Rev. of Microbiology*.
121. Sokal, R. R. 1974. Classifications: purposes, principles, progress, and prospects. *Science*. 185: 1115-1123.
122. Stonebreaker, M. 1980. Retrospection on a data base system. *Trans. Database Systems*. 5.
123. Szasz, T. S. 1972. *The Myth of Mental Illness*. London: Paladin.
124. Szolovits, P., and S. G. Pauker. 1979. Computers and clinical decision making: whether, how, and for whom? *Proc. IEEE.* 67: 1224-1226.
125. Temkin, O. 1968. The history of classification in the medical sciences. *The Role and Methodology of Classification in Psychiatry and Psychopathology*. U.S. Department of Health, Education,

and Welfare, U.S. Public Health Service, Bull. 1584.

126. ———. 1945. *The Falling Sickness.* Baltimore: Johns Hopkins University Press.

127. ———. 1963. *The Scientific Approach to Disease: Specific Entity and Individual Sickness.* Edited by C. C. Crombe. New York: Basic Books.

128. Tribus, M., and E. C. McIrvine. 1971. Energy and information. *Sci. Amer.* 225: 188.

129. Turing, A. M. 1956. Can machines think? *The World of Mathematics.* Edited by J. R. Newman. New York: Simon and Schuster.

130. Tversky, A. 1979. First Ann. Meeting of the Cognitive Science Society. La Jolla, Ca.

131. Warner, H. R. 1979. *Computer-Assisted Medical Decision Making.* New York: Academic Press.

132. Warner, H. R., A. F. Toronto, L. G. Veasey, and R. Stephenson. 1961. A mathematical approach to medical diagnosis. *Jour. Amer. Med. Assoc.* 177: 177-182.

133. Wasserman, A. I., and S. Gutz. 1982. The future of programming. *Comm. of the ACM.* 25: 196-206.

134. Weed, L. 1969. *Medical Records, Medical Education and Patient Care.* Cleveland: The Press of Case Western Reserve University.

135. Weizenbaum, J. 1976. *Computer Power and Human Reason.* San Francisco: Freeman.

136. Whitehead, A. N. 1920. *The Concept of Nature.* Cambridge, England: Cambridge University Press.

137. ———. 1938. *Modes of Thought.* New York: The Macmillan Company.

138. Whittemore, B. J., and M. C. Yovits. 1974. A generalized concept for the analysis of information. *Information Science: Search for Identity.* Edited by A. Debons. New York: Marcel-Dekker (pp. 29-45).

139. Wilson, E. B. 1925. *The cell in development and heredity* (3d ed.). New York: The Macmillan Company.

140. Winograd, T. 1972. *Understanding Natural Language.* New York: Academic Press.

141. Zadeh, L. A. 1976. The concept of a linguistic variable and its application to approximate reasoning. *Inform. Sci.* 9: 43-80.

142. ———. 1977. A fuzzy algorithmic approach to the definition of complex or imprecise concepts. *Int. Jour. Man-Machine Studies.* 8: 249-291.

143. ———. 1978. PRUF - a meaning representation language for natural languages. *Int. Jour. Man-Machine Studies.* 10: 395-460.

Index

Designer: UC Press Staff
Compositor: Janet Sheila Brown
Printer: Edwards Brothers
Binder: Edwards Brothers
Text: 11/13 English Times
Display: English Times